SOCIOLOGY IN ACTION

INVESTIGATING HEALTH, WELFARE AND POVERTY

PAUL TROWLER

UNWIN HYMAN

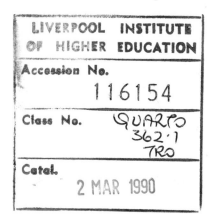
Published in 1989 by
Unwin Hyman Limited
15/17 Broadwick Street
London WIV IFP

British Library Cataloguing in Publication Data

Trowler, Paul
  Investigating health, welfare and poverty.—
  (Sociology in action).
  1. Great Britain. Social policies
  I. Title   II. Series
  361.6'1'0941

  ISBN 0–04–448040–7

Cover by Oxford Illustrators
Designed by Bob Wright
Cartoons by David Simonds

Typeset by August Filmsetting, Haydock, St Helens
Printed in Great Britain by Scotprint Ltd, Musselburgh

Contents

Introduction

The *Sociology in Action* series aims to provide readers with an interesting and up-to-date account of the main themes in the areas it covers. The series has been written primarily for students following the sociology 'A' and 'AS' – level syllabus. However, it is also designed to be helpful to those entering for GCSE examinations in Sociology, as well as related disciplines. To this end, each book relates the issues specific to its subject area to the broader concerns of social science and the humanities. The philosophy underlying the series has been to encourage students to deepen their understanding of the subject by engaging in short exercises and larger-scale projects as they progress through the books. The authors have followed the student-centred approach which is the basis of good teaching and learning.

Investigating Health, Welfare and Poverty provides a factual account of the state of Britain's health, the welfare services and the extent of poverty. It also introduces students to the important debates around these issues, both within Sociology as an academic discipline and in the contemporary political arena. At the same time, the book deepens students' understanding of the broader sociological concerns, such as the sociology of stratification, women, and ethnic minorities, through the analysis of health and welfare—related topics in these areas.

The book includes exercises and projects which, it is hoped, will be developed and modified according to the aims and needs of the students and the facilities available. The book was written primarily from a sociological perspective but with the aims of other courses in mind. These include those in the health and welfare field validated by BTEC, and professional courses with a sociological component in this field. Students following such courses will find the suggested exercises and projects included here useful in making final decisions about their assessed assignments, and, hopefully, will take up the invitation offered by the book to become actively involved in the study of health, welfare and poverty.

Paul Trowler

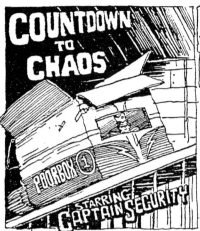

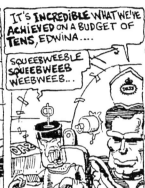

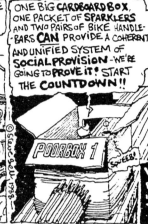

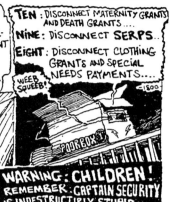

☐ **Before reading further, note down the areas connected to health that you think sociologists (as opposed to medics or psychologists) would address themselves to. After glancing through the table of contents, the chapters themselves and the index, compare the areas that are dealt with and your prediction. Are there any differences—extra areas or omissions?**

This chapter aims to set the scene for the rest of the book. In it we will examine some of the concepts used in the study of (in turn) health, welfare and poverty.

Health

The nature of 'health'

The World Health Organisation defines health as:

> 'Not the mere absence of disease, but total physical, mental and social well-being'.

Unfortunately, this is so vague as to be almost useless. In practice the medical profession (and the population at large) tend to define health in a *negative* way:

> 'The condition in which there is an absence of disease or disability'.

This raises some problems too, mainly concerned with identifying when a disease is or is not present.

The distinction between having a disease rather than just being 'off-colour', 'not on top form' etc is unclear. The following process must occur before we are identified officially as having a disease:
recognition (of bodily events as symptoms of disease by the individual);
definition (of the symptoms as serious enough to take to the doctor);
action (specifically, of going to the doctor).

Only at this point is there an 'official' definition of ill-health, which may lead to further action such as hospitalisation, being prescribed a medicine or being given time off work. Doctors refer to the 'clinical iceberg'—they only see those who present themselves to them and not the large proportion who are 'below the waves'—ie not presented.

The clinical iceberg

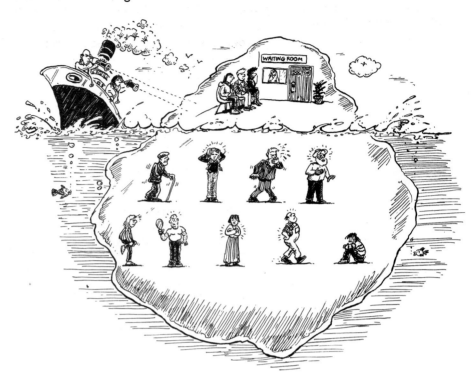

□ **Individually, brainstorm the factors which influence the decision to go to the doctors with an illness (include both 'pushing' and 'pulling' factors, ie those which impel you to go, and those which make you not want to).**

In plenary, collate your ideas. What sociological insights does the resulting list give you about the clinical iceberg?

Two week incidence of symptoms and subsequent behaviour in a random sample of 1000 adults living in London.

*Individuals with symptoms taking no action	188
*Individuals with symptoms taking non-medical action	562
GP patients	168
Hospital out-patients	28
Hospital in-patients	5
Total (including 49 in sample with no symptoms—ie healthy)	1000

Source: Wadsworth *et al*, 1971, (in G. Scambler, *Illness Behaviour*, in M. Morgan *et al*, *Sociological Approaches to Health and Medicine*), Croom Helm, London 1985, p 43.

We can't identify a 'normal' state, deviation from which counts as disease. This is because people's bodies are so different. In fact most of us put up with many symptoms for much of the time without ever going through the processes of recognition, definition and action. At any one time around 56 per cent of men and 70 per cent of women feel unwell in some way or have a recurring health problem. Yet men visit their doctor only three times a year, and women four times (on average).

Consequently, what counts as 'illness' differs between cultures and in history. What counts as 'health' must be socially constructed and is therefore variable, too.

The nature of 'disease'

While 'illness' refers to the subjective feeling of 'not being well', the more specific term 'disease' refers to the medically diagnosed condition

□ **Measures of the level of ill-health are available (infant mortality rate, expectation of life etc) but no measure of *health*. This has been an obstacle to the World Health Organisation's *Health For All* campaign—its success cannot be measured. Is it possible to develop a measure of health so that general improvements in it nationally could be quantified? If so, what form/s might it take?**

□ **Give an example of the reverse; someone who is ill, but does not have a 'disease'.**

which has given rise to signs and symptoms in a patient. It is therefore possible to have no 'illness', yet have a disease. An example of this is people with symptomless ('asymptomatic') high blood pressure ('hypertension'). They are not ill, but they have a disease.

The following are the 17 categories of diseases identified by the World Health Organisation:

Category of disease	Examples
1. Infections and parasitic diseases	malaria, viral hepatitis
2. Neoplasms	Hodgkin's disease, malignant neoplasm of the larynx
3. Endocrine, nutritional and metabolic diseases and immunity disorders	diabetes mellitus, gout
4. Diseases of blood and blood-forming organs	iron-deficiency anaemia, diseases of white blood cells
5. Mental disorders	alcohol-dependence syndrome, physical symptoms of mental disorder
6. Diseases of the nervous system and sense organs	epilepsy, migraine
7. Diseases of the circulatory system	hypertension, acute myocardial infarction
8. Diseases of the respiratory system	asbestosis, acute sinusitis
9. Diseases of the digestive system	appendicitis
10. Diseases of the genitourinary system	renal failure, female infertility
11. Complications of childbirth and pregnancy	excessive vomiting in pregnancy
12. Diseases of the skin and subcutaneous tissue	dermatitis, psoriasis
13. Diseases of the musculoskeletal system and connective tissue	rheumatoid arthritis
14. Congenital anomalies	spina bifida, cleft palate
15. Certain conditions originating in the perinatal period (ie just prior to and soon after birth)	slow fetal growth, birth trauma
16. Symptoms, signs and ill-defined conditions	symptoms involving head and neck, sudden death—cause unknown
17. Injury and poisoning	fracture of carpal bone, poisoning by psychotropic drugs

□ **In which category would the following diseases go ... AIDS, schizophrenia, asthma, stomach cancer, stomach ulcers?**

Source: WHO, *International Classification of Diseases*, Geneva 1977 (ninth edition)

Doctors are concerned to establish the aetiology of a disease, ie its causes. This can best be established through large-scale epidemiological studies of its incidence. For example the link between cigarette smoking and lung cancer was discovered in the following way:

1 Doctors noticed that among patients with lung cancer, smokers outnumbered non-smokers.

2 A survey was carried out among lung-cancer sufferers, and this confirmed the correlation between smoking and the disease (though this did not necessarily mean smoking *caused* it, merely that the two were often found together).

3 Finally, work in the laboratory demonstrated that elements in cigarettes could cause cancer in animals, and the mechanism by which this occurred was identified.

☐ **Choose any of the individuals named in this chart and research their contribution to the development of medicine.**

Other terms commonly used in the study of disease are morbidity and mortality. Morbidity refers to ill-health resulting from disease, mortality to death. The mortality rate is the number of deaths in a given year and place per 1000 of the population.

Some important developments in medicine

History of medicine timechart

Years	Eras	Individuals		Events and trends
10,000BC 3,000BC	Prehistoric	None that we know about		Belief in magic—charms, spells, etc. Primitive surgery—trephinning. Use of plants, roots and berries as medicines. Ideas about medicine limited by supernatural view of world. Problem for historians of no written evidence.
	Egyptian	Imhotep		*Egyptians*—superstition mixed with a more scientific approach. Use of drugs and preservatives—embalming. Very aware of hygiene—washed frequently. Settled way of life helped ideas to develop and they were written down. Religious beliefs stopped them using dissection, so they knew little about how the body worked.
	Chinese	Asclepios Hippocrates		*Greeks*—strong supernatural beliefs but believed in hygiene and fitness. Philosophers and doctors studied the human body at Alexandria where dissection was permitted. Beginnings of medical schools.
400BC	Greek Babylonian Indian			*China*—discoveries made here long before Europe. Use of acupuncture. *India*—skilled surgeons. *Babylon*—one of the first cities to have public health facilities.
400AD	Roman	Galen		Importance of public health—sewers, drains, aqueducts and public baths. Military hospitals. Spread of Empire meant spread of ideas. Large number of unqualified doctors meant that most were distrusted.
1500AD	Dark Ages and Middle Ages	Avicenna Rhazes Albicasis		Little progress in medicine in Europe due to fall of Roman Empire and influence of Church which believed that disease was a punishment from God. Black Death. Arab Empire—centre of medicine. Growth of medical schools—Salerno and Cairo.
1700AD	Renaiss-ance	Vesalius Paré Harvey	Paracelsus Sydenham	Increase in books and travel encourages spread of ideas. Study of anatomy becomes more common. Much greater awareness of causes of disease and way the body works.
1900AD	18th and 19th Centuries	Jenner Pasteur Simpson Lister Semmelweis Nightingale	Koch Chadwick Freud	Industrial Revolution—growth of towns leads to overcrowding. Public Health Acts in Britain (1848 & 75) passed to improve sanitation and prevent the spread of disease. Growth of hospitals. Improvements in nursing. Rapid progress in all areas of medicine in 19th century—understanding of germs, use of chloroform in surgery, vaccination, etc.
2000AD	20th Century	Ehrlich Manson Fleming Barnard		Much greater understanding of disease and its treatment including syphilis, TB, diphtheria and malaria. National Health Service and growth of Welfare State in Britain. World wars lead to improvements in drugs, surgery and the fight against disease. World Health Organisation—spread of health education and prevention of disease in Third World. Use of high technology in Western hospitals.

Source: L. Hartley, *The History of Medicine*, Basil Blackwell.

The NHS Today

In 1985, the NHS cost in the region of £16·5 billion a year to run. It has, in recent years, been the subject of considerable criticism and subsequent reorganisation. From 1948 to 1974, responsibility for the nation's health was shared by:

Regional Hospital Boards (hospitals);
Local Authorities (ambulance, home health support services etc);
Local Executive Councils (GPs and other services).

This tripartite structure caused considerable administrative headaches and was criticised for being a particularly expensive form of management. Beveridge had believed that the costs of the NHS would fall as a result of the improved health of a nation under its care. Instead, costs rose each year.

In 1974 the NHS was reorganised so that the vast majority of the services were under the control of (in order of diminishing size) Regional Health Authorities, Area Health Authorities and local District Management Teams. A new complaints procedure was set up. In each district there was (and still is) a Community Health Council, which monitors the running of the district's health services and receives complaints from the public. CHCs have been criticised for being ineffective and comprising of mainly middle class members who are out of touch with the health problems of ordinary people. Another means of complaint about health services is through the NHS Ombudsman, also established in 1974. Once again, the limited powers of this office mean that there is little faith in its effectiveness.

☐ **The 'phone number and address of your local CHC is in the 'phone book. They will be happy to tell you about their work (this is part of their function). Find as much information about them as you can and make a presentation to the group you are studying with. A similar exercise can be done for the NHS Ombudsman. The address to write to is:**

The Health Service Commissioner for England, Church House, Great Smith Street, London, SW1P 3BW.

One way of judging the effectiveness of measures for the redress of grievance is the number of people in the population who are aware of the existence of CHCs and know how to call upon their services. Develop a means of quantifying this.

☐ **Which Health District are you in? (The bar chart on page 65 has a list of them.)**

Again, however, this structure was felt to be inefficient and ineffective. By 1983 the Area Health Authorities had been abolished, their functions now being carried out by reorganised District Health Authorities. The structure now is shown in Table 1 on page 10.

The Health Services Supervisory Board, (which makes decisions about overall objectives and resources), and the full-time NHS Management Board (which plan how the former's policies will be put into effect) have existed only since 1985. The Management Board has a chairman who is, in effect, the managing director of the NHS. Locally, too, single General Managers have been put in charge, replacing the old consensus style management.

Table I: Levels of administration of the NHS (UK)

Population served		Number of units
56 million	Parliament	I
56 million	Department of Health (with some of its functions being performed by their respective Offices in Scotland, Wales and Northern Ireland)	I
56 million	Health Services Supervisory Board	I
56 million	NHS Management Board	I
I–5 million	Regional Health Authorities	17
100,000–500,000	District Health Authorities	221
100,000–500,000	Community Health Councils	221
50,000–500,000	Family Practitioner Committees	100
2,000–20,000	GP units (practices)	9,000 (about)

On 31 January 1989 the Government announced what Health Secretary Kenneth Clarke referred to as 'the most formidable programme of reform in the history of the NHS'. The discussion document, a White Paper called *Working For Patients* (HMSO, CMND 555) made the following proposals:

- That many hospitals should become self-governing and should sell services to doctors, health authorities, private patients and other hospitals. They would be given resources by the NHS, though these would reflect the ability of hospitals to attract patients.
- That many doctors should be given more financial responsibility by being given their own funds to administer, and targets of cost-effectiveness to meet (failure to do so would result in financial penalties). Costs of prescribed drugs, for example, would be carefully monitored in each practice. Again, funds from the NHS would be related to doctor's 'attractiveness' to patients. Doctors would be allowed to advertise.
- That DHAs should become more like agencies; not providing health services but buying them from hospitals and doctors for patients. Management at all levels of the NHS (RHAs, DHAs, FPCs) would become more like that of businesses, with a general manager and finance director. Local authorities and health professionals would lose much of their representation on these bodies.
- Cost-effectiveness throughout the system would be carefully monitored by auditors (accountants) and all parts of it (including the previously powerful consultants) would be answerable to management for lack of efficiency or effectiveness.

These developments should not be seen in isolation. They mirror very closely Government policy in other fields which are under its direct control. Local authorities have been 'rate capped' and had grants to them reduced as a punishment for 'over-spending' in much the same way as will happen to doctors and hospitals. The civil service has already seen financial responsibility devolved to the local level and efficiencies introduced under the *Financial Management Initiative*. Some areas of the civil service will become autonomous bodies in the near future, just like the hospitals under these proposals. Finally, the 1988 Education Act allows schools to become autonomous (and to compete for pupils), as well as giving them control over finances rather than their Local Education Authorities.

☐ **Individually, compile a list of all the voluntary welfare organisations you can think of. In groups, collate the lists. Choose any organisation, and, in pairs, research its history and current work. Identify which are active in your area. Addresses can be found in *The Charities Digest* and from the Volunteer Centre (see bibliography).**

Welfare

The 'Welfare State'

A Welfare State can be defined as:

> 'a state with a democratic form of government which assumes responsibility for the well-being of its citizens through a range of interventions in the market economy'.

The term Welfare State includes both the ideas of state responsibility for welfare, and the institutions and practices through which this idea is realised. By market economy we mean:

> 'an economy in which enterprise is in private hands and operates on the basis of the search for profit'.

Market economies are contrasted to command economies, where the state controls (and usually owns) the means of production.

There is a common misconception that the Welfare State began in the 1945–1951 period of post-war Labour Government. In fact, as the time chart below shows, its history is much longer than that. However, the structure of the modern Welfare State and many of the principles operating today were established then, following the recommendations of the Beveridge Report on *National Insurance and Allied Services, 1942*. Beveridge identified 'five giants' which it was the duty of the state to tackle and eliminate. They were:

Idleness (unemployment)   Squalor (poor housing)
Disease (poor health)   Want (poverty)
Ignorance (lack of education)

☐ **Beveridge concentrated on these five areas for social policy in his report. Other areas of government intervention which could be considered part of the welfare state are listed below. Which do you include and exclude as part of the Welfare State?**

> **Services for old people (eg old people's homes)**
> **Tax relief for mortgages and dependents ('fiscal social security')**
> **Refuse collection**
> **Services for gypsies and vagrants**
> **Social work**
> **Environmental protection**
> **Employment services**
> **Planning services**
> **Probation and after-care service for offenders**
> **Services for children and young people**
> **Transport services (roads, buses, rail)**
> **Leisure services (leisure centres, swimming pools)**
> **Job perks: free membership of BUPA, pension, car etc ('occupational social security'—these are partly funded by the state through tax relief)**

☐ **Identify three commercial organisations involved in the provision of welfare services.**

The state and welfare in Britain

There are three ways in which the state can be involved in welfare. These are:

- provision of services directly (eg benefits from the DSS);
- subsidy of services. The Training Commission, later to become the Training Agency, which funds voluntary organisations, is an important example here—£285 million to Community Programme schemes in 1983/4;
- regulation of services (eg legislation on rented housing).

The following chart summarises the history of the welfare state as far as the statutory sector is concerned.

Table 2:   The history of the welfare state

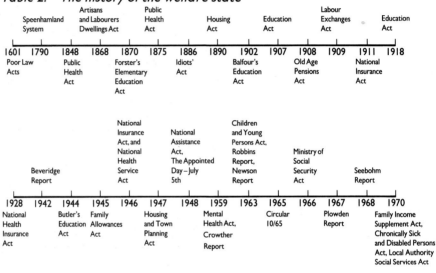

Above	Speenhamland System		Artisans and Labourers Dwellings Act		Public Health Act			Housing Act		Education Act		Labour Exchanges Act		Education Act
Year	1601	1790	1848	1868	1870	1875	1886	1890	1902	1907	1908	1909	1911	1918
Below	Poor Law Acts		Public Health Act		Forster's Elementary Education Act		Idiots' Act		Balfour's Education Act		Old Age Pensions Act		National Insurance Act	

Above		Beveridge Report			National Insurance Act, and National Health Service Act		National Assistance Act, The Appointed Day – July 5th		Children and Young Persons Act, Robbins Report, Newson Report		Ministry of Social Security Act		Seebohm Report	
Year	1928	1942	1944	1945	1946	1947	1948	1959	1963	1965	1966	1967	1968	1970
Below	National Health Insurance Act		Butler's Education Act	Family Allowances Act		Housing and Town Planning Act		Mental Health Act, Crowther Report		Circular 10/65		Plowden Report		Family Income Supplement Act, Chronically Sick and Disabled Persons Act, Local Authority Social Services Act

Above	Housing Finance Act		Health and Safety at Work Act			Education Act	Budget tax cuts (esp for higher rate-payers). Increase in VAT		Social Security and Housing Benefits Act		Abolition of Domestic Rates (Scotland) Act	
Year	1972	1973	1974	1975	1976	1977	1979	1980	1982	1986	1987	1988
Below		NHS Reorganisation Act		Child Benefit Act, Social Security (Pensions) Act		Housing (Homeless Persons) Act		Social Security Acts, Education Act		Social Security Act		Social Security Act, Education Reform Act

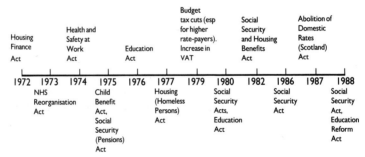

☐ **Choose any one of the reports or Acts of Parliament referred to here and research it. Use the references listed in the bibliography to help you. Report back to the group you are studying with when you've finished.**

However the state is only one of the providers of welfare services. The Wolfenden Report (*The Future of Voluntary Organisations*) identified four sectors which can provide social services and health care:

- statutory (organisations set up by legislation in parliament);
- voluntary (non-statutory organisations, often charities);
- commercial (profit-making businesses), and;
- informal (relatives, neighbours and friends).

In Britain we have a combination of these four sectors, a situation which the Wolfenden Report called 'welfare pluralism'. The Conservative governments since 1979 have attempted to alter the mix of this pluralism, reducing the traditionally strong role of the state and increasing the role of the other three sectors. The reasons for this are, in summary, a belief that:

- state organisations are 'captured' by professionals who use them in their own interests, not those of clients;
- state services are expensive and bureaucratic compared to other forms of provision. Private schemes and charitable agencies give more choice and efficiency than state schemes;
- state organisations are too large and unresponsive to the needs and wishes of clients, and as a result people no longer support them;
- generally, state intervention in society should be reduced so that people become more responsible for themselves and their families (a reduction of the role of the 'nanny state' and its attendant 'dependency culture', to use Mrs Thatcher's terms);
- compulsory insurance, state programmes etc belong to the pre-war and early post-war eras, they are out of date in modern society;
- the strategy of equality (ie redistributing resources from the rich to the poor through welfare benefits and services) has gone far enough, probably too far;
- the costs of the Welfare State are too great—demand is unlimited and there are constantly rising expectations;
- government action has unintended consequences—eg the importance of the family declines, people become unwilling to undertake low wage labour, incentives to succeed are reduced;
- government has become overloaded—the system is too complex and outcomes are no longer predictable;
- government spending on welfare is counter-productive—it creates inflation which only causes further problems;
- governments act according to the 'vote-motive', ie they offer welfare goodies as a bribe for election or re-election. This means that welfare services are set up irresponsibly, without thought to cost or consequences.

☐ **What are the particular *advantages* of a) commercial, b) voluntary and c) informal provision of services?**

■ **The following are the possible different relationships between the four sectors of welfare provision. Under each one, give an example of a service which falls under this category in Britain and the sector or sectors which provide it (for example, under 'sole provider' would come social clubs for the elderly or handicapped provided by voluntary organisations such as Help the Aged).**

Sole provider   Temporary relief   Complementary   Competitive

Funding the Welfare State

The NHS in particular has been plagued by questions of funding; how much should be spent on it, and how far patients should be asked to contribute to expenses (eg by prescription charges and 'hotel bills' for staying in hospital). Similar sorts of questions have surrounded the issue of welfare benefits; how generous should they be, how shall 'scroungers' be rooted out, should they go only to the most needy, and so on. Such questions became particularly important with the decline of the British economy in the early 1970s and the subsequent economic problems this created. Though, arguably, the economy has now recovered, funding is still at the root of a crisis that has affected the welfare state in the 1980s. There are a number of aspects to this crisis:

ps, develop
als to recommend
to government four ways
in which demand for
medical treatment can be
limited. You might
consider (among other
things); means testing,
introducing charges for
some things, need
testing, excluding some
services from the NHS
altogether (if so which?),
trying to get non-state
institutions to share the
financial burden, and
encouraging people to
opt out of the Welfare
State altogether.

☐ 'The Government have
already increased
spending (on the NHS)
from £7·75 billion in
1978–79 to £18·75 billion
this year.' (Norman
Fowler, Secretary of
State for Social Services,
DHSS press release,
September 1986.)

What else would we need
to know to be able to test
the claim that this shows
that the government has
funded an increase in the
quantity and quality of
NHS services?

- The government's desire to cut public expenditure means that the funding of the Welfare State receives little government enthusiasm, indeed it is seen as a barrier to recovery and prosperity.
- The government's desire to cut taxes means that there are inadequate funds for health and welfare services.
- There has been a public loss of confidence in the idea of a Welfare State, which has affected attitudes to it, both inside and outside its institutions.
- Demographic factors have not helped; an increasingly ageing population places greater financial burdens on health and social services.
- Medical treatment is becoming more expensive, as it increasingly involves high technology and expensive drugs. It therefore demands an ever higher proportion of state expenditure.
- As medical expertise becomes greater, and the potential for curative medicine improves, demand increases. If access to medical services is easy and free or cheap there is potentially unlimited demand (particularly in view of the flexible way in which 'ill-health' is defined and the changing definitions of 'normal health'). Left alone, the medical profession would want to increase the resources available to it to meet this demand. There would be a spiral in expenditure which would lead to severe economic problems nationally. The government's responsibility, therefore, is to draw the line at which the welfare state has a responsibility to meet need.

Conservative governments of the early 80s have maintained that the Welfare State is safe in their hands, indeed that the funding of it has increased since the last Labour government left office in 1979. However this is debatable.

Poverty

Chapter 3 will discuss the problems associated with defining 'poverty', so here we will concentrate on examining the changing attitudes towards poverty in Britain.

The earliest official responses to poverty began with the Poor Law Acts of the early seventeenth century. Parishes (and, after 1782 'Unions'—combinations of parishes), provided relief for orphans, the sick and the aged. Workhouses were run for the able-bodied poor. Some of these were privately run (receiving a fee from the parishes for the poor they accepted) and conditions in them were very bad. In these early days the attitude towards the poor was that if they were able-bodied 'sturdy beggars' then their poverty was the result of indolence or some other personal failing.

In 1795 there was the beginning of a change in this attitude. Some of those in positions of power began to appreciate that poverty could be caused by inadequate wages and unemployment, resulting from factors which the individual worker had no control over. A system of poor relief known as the Speenhamland System began in that year in Berkshire, and quickly spread around central and southern England. It gave a supplement to the wages of workers who had large families and whose income was inadequate. It was also 'index linked', in that the amount of income-supplement given depended upon the price of bread at the time.

Of the numerous problems connected to the Speenhamland System, the one that most exercised the minds of those in power was its cost. The 'poor rate' (the tax collected to pay for relief of the poor) increased dramatically with its introduction. It was primarily this that led to the Poor Law Amendment Act of 1834. This marked a return to the view that poverty was the fault of the poor persons who (unless they were orphans, sick or old) should be punished. The able-bodied poor were no longer eligible for 'outdoor relief' and had to enter workhouses. These were deliberately kept as unpleasant as possible in accordance with the principle of 'less eligibility'—ie entering a workhouse was made much less attractive than even the worst kind of employment outside. This had the desired result; many people declined to accept 'indoor relief'. In times of unemployment this had the effect of creating much poverty and misery. The authorities, though, believed it was forcing the idle to work.

The new Poor Law of 1834 continued to operate virtually unchanged until 1908. However, there was again a swing in attitudes towards the poor which partly resulted from the studies of poverty by Booth and Rowntree (see pages 42–43). Again, it was realised that involuntary unemployment and low wages could cause poverty just as much as sickness and old age, and that poverty was an economic problem, not a moral one. A new set of legislation began to be implemented which gradually replaced the Poor Law. Old age pensions were introduced (for some) in 1908, while limited health and unemployment insurance was set up by the government in 1911. These were the foundations of the modern Welfare State, which was mainly constructed between 1945 and 1950 following the Beveridge Report of 1942.

It is arguably the case that attitudes are now swinging back to those which motivated the passing of the 1834 Poor Law Amendment Act. Again, the view that the principle cause of poverty is the ignorance and idleness of the poor themselves seems to have become the dominant one. Once again this has been encapsulated in legislation. The 1986 Social Security Act (which came into operation in 1988) has been called the most important social welfare measure since the post-war legislation which followed the Beveridge Report. This Act introduced the following measures:

- It replaced Supplementary Benefit with Income Support (both being non-contributory and means-tested). As a result, the level of benefit for many was reduced (particularly for the young), benefit was cut entirely in some cases (for example young people who moved away from their families without good reason), and discretionary payments for cases of special hardship were removed.
- It set up the Social Fund, partly to help those cases of special hardship now not covered by Income Support. However:
  - almost all payments are loans, not (as before) grants;
  - they do not *have* to be paid—the Government can decide;
  - there is only a limited amount in Social Fund each year;
  - claimants in a financial crisis must try elsewhere for money first;
  - appeals will not be to independent bodies but to the DSS.
- It replaced Family Income Supplement with Family Credit, which in

some ways is more generous but may not be claimed by many of those eligible for it (family heads in work but on low incomes).

● It reduced the amount of state pension for those retiring early next century, by limiting the link between earnings now and pension then. At the same time the Act made it easier and cheaper to take out private pensions (though with these there is no guarantee what the eventual pension will be).

Other legislative measures concerning poverty have consolidated this new approach. The 1988 Social Security Act withdrew benefits from most people under 18. Its assumption was that young people should either be in jobs or accept a place on the Youth Training Scheme. One TUC official said of this measure:

> 'We are heading for a new Dickensian era where instead of little match girls we have drug addicts and child prostitutes'.
> (*The Independent*, 28 December 1988.)

It was estimated that at least 14,000 people between the ages of 16 and 17 were without jobs or income during Christmas 1988.

☐ **Other Conservative social security measures of recent years include the following. Explain them in terms of the New Right philosophy (outlined on pages 22–24).**

- **The failure to increase Child Benefit in line with inflation in some years (Child Benefit is a universal benefit, it is paid to all mothers with more than one child).**
- **An increase in prescription charges (from 20p in 1979) and charges introduced for dental checks and eyes tests.**
- **After 1982 local education authorities were not obliged to provide school meals (except for some benefit claimants) or nursery education.**
- **The council house building programme was stopped or cut in a number of years.**
- **Resources for the DSS to identify fraudulent claimants were greatly increased.**
- **Income tax was reduced dramatically between 1979 and 1988, most of the benefit going to higher rate taxpayers (maximum level was cut to 60 per cent).**
- **Domestic rates were abolished and replaced by the poll tax, initially only in Scotland. Previously, rates charges increased with the more land you owned and the bigger and better your house. Poll tax is a flat-rate charged on individuals, regardless of any property they own.**

The effect of the social security changes has been to leave 80 per cent of the poorest claimants worse off than they were before April 1988 and to intensify the poverty trap. A study of 30,000 people who consulted the Citizens Advice Bureaux in May 1988 was conducted by that organisation. Its main findings were:

- stricter means tests meant higher rates of non-claiming;
- some claimants who took a job found themselves worse off as the amount of work people could do and still claim Income Support was cut from 30 hours to 24 hours;

- people in work and claiming Family Credit were frequently worse off because their mortgage interest payments were no longer made for them;
- single parents in work and claiming benefit found their child care and work expense payments cut;
- grants for tools and clothing to help people start work were no longer available;
- benefits were no longer payable during the first two weeks of work;
- cuts in housing benefit left the majority worse off;
- compensation for the loss of free school meals was inadequate, again leaving claimants worse off.

☐ **'The purpose of Newspeak was not only to provide a medium of expression for the world-view and mental habits proper to the [the inhabitants of that country] ... but to make all other modes of thought impossible. It was intended that ... a heretical thought ... should be literally unthinkable... Its vocabulary was so constructed as to give exact and often very subtle expression to every meaning that a Party member could properly wish to express, while excluding all other meanings....'**

Source: G. Orwell, *Nineteen Eighty-Four*, Secker and Warburg, London 1949, pp 305–6

☐ **ESSAY**

'What counts as illness and health differs both historically and geographically'. Explain this statement and discuss the problems it poses both for sociologists and for medics.

Very often, terms generated by the government in the field of social welfare seem to have the characteristics of Newspeak. 'Community care' is a good example; the word 'community' suggests a warm, strong and cooperative group, 'care' evokes very positive associations. In the past the terms used in welfare policy were not so carefully constructed. The following are some examples of now outmoded terms:

'National Assistance' 'Family Allowance' 'Rent and Rate Rebates' 'Labour Exchange'

Compile a list of modern welfare policy terms (particularly the names of types of social security benefits) and comment on the connotations they have.

Bibliography

Alcock, P. *Poverty and State Support*, Longman, London 1987

Allsop, J. *Health Policy and the NHS*, Longman, London 1984

Barker, P. (ed) *The Founders of the Welfare State*, Heinemann, London 1984

Baugh, W. E. *Introduction to the Social Services*, Macmillan, London 1987

Beveridge, W. *Social Insurance and Allied Services*, HMSO Cmd 6404, London 1942, reprinted 1984

Brenton, M. and Ungerson, C. *The Yearbook of Social Policy*, Longman (annually—check for the most recent edition)

Brenton, M. *The Voluntary Sector in British Social Services*, Longman, London 1985

Charities Digest. Published annually by The Family Welfare Association

Committee of Inquiry into the Future Development of the Public Health Function, *Public Health in England*, HMSO, London 1988

Graham, H. *Health and Welfare*, Macmillan, London 1985

Ham, C. *Health Policy in Britain*, Macmillan, London 1985 (second edition)

Johnson, N. *The Welfare State in Transition*, Wheatsheaf Books, Brighton 1987

Mays, J. *Penelope Hall's Social Services of England and Wales*, RKP, London 1983 (check for the most recent edition)

Mishra, R. *The Welfare State in Crisis*, Wheatsheaf Books, Brighton 1984

Papadakis, E. and Taylor-Gooby, P. *The Private Provision of Public Welfare*, Wheatsheaf Books, Brighton 1987

Thane, P. *The Foundations of the Welfare State*, Longman, London 1982

Trowler, P. and Riley, M. *Topics in Sociology*, Unwin Hyman, London 1984

Trowler, P. *Further Topics in Sociology*, Unwin Hyman, London 1985

Watkin, B. *Documents on Health and Social Services—1824 to the Present Day*, Methuen, London 1975

Wolfenden, J. *The Future of Voluntary Organisations*, Croom Helm, London 1978

The volunteer centre is the national advisory agency on volunteer and community involvement. Its address is 29 Lower Kings Rd., Berkhamsted, Herts, HP4 2QB, (04427) 73311

2 · Approaching the study of health and welfare

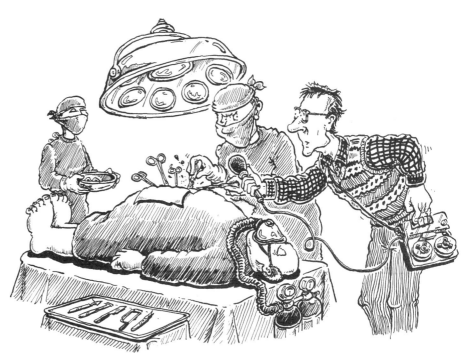

"And how many patients do you lose in this sort of operation, Doctor?"

The perspectives

This chapter will first examine some of the important perspectives on the issues of health, welfare and poverty. These are phenomenology, interactionism, the New Right, the Social Democrats, Functionalism, Marxism and Feminism. Secondly it will outline the research methods available to students interested in these issues. The chapter aims to go beyond a focus on health, welfare and poverty, however, to address general issues such as the connections between perspectives and their preferred methods, the drawbacks and advantages of particular methods, and questions of objectivity in research.

The phenomenological perspective

From a phenomenological perspective the first thing to do when researching issues of health, welfare and poverty is to dispense with preconceptions. Events must be treated as 'strange'—the researcher should refuse to participate in the shared meanings which underlie all social interaction. Doing this enables her/him to uncover the nature of those meanings (which are normally so obvious to the participants that they are not conscious of their presence). The researcher, then, behaves like a Martian, seeing human interaction for the first time; s/he is free of any of the influences of socialisation.

The phenomenological perspective in sociology argues that:

- the social world has no objective existence, its reality is nothing more than the shared meanings and beliefs we have about it
- these meanings seem so obvious to the members of a society that they do not notice them; they are taken for granted
- the task of the sociologist is to uncover these meanings, not in an attempt to establish any scientific laws or universal truths about social behaviour but to show how particular small social systems work.

For example, what is 'common sense' to an Australian aborigine is completely alien to a British person, and vice versa. The two are living in completely different worlds. These worlds have been and are being constructed for them and by them in the course of their social interaction. While this may clearly be true in the aborigine/British example, it is also true for closer cultures (France/Italy) and for groups within one culture (civil servants in London/young unemployed in Glasgow).

Anthropologists (students of 'simple' societies) use this sort of method in their studies. They usually come from cultures which are radically different from the ones they are studying, so for them it is easier. However their training and experience makes them good at using 'ethnomethodology' (as this approach is called) in their own cultures too. An example of its use in the study of health comes from a book called *Medical Encounters*. Its editors say:

'We asked our contributors to treat their own experiences [of illness and health care] as "strange" and to prepare an account of how they attempted to produce order out of these experiences ...' (page 10).

For one of the contributors, anthropologist Rosemary Firth who was admitted to a tropical diseases hospital after fieldwork in Malaysia, the experience was an excellent opportunity to observe the NHS as she would a tribe in the Far East ...

'... at 4.00 pm nurses in white uniforms (?lowest grade) came round with trolleys ... At 8.15 pm hot drinks were brought round. When we were all safely in bed, a nurse (white uniform, no belt buckle) looked in to ask if anyone wanted a sleeping tablet ... After tea at 6.00 am, and breakfast in bed about 7.30 am, a flock of activities and routines to be noted. Pulse, temperature, weighing, blood samples taken, instructions about preserving specimens given; a series of people in different coloured overalls bring in instruments for cleaning—dusting, polishing and so on. Green overalls bring food and clean. Pink overalls seem to take away the pans and dusters.' (pp 114–115.)

☐ **Write a similar account of a consultation you've had with a GP. Pay special attention to the symbols of office, the stages of the consultation, who spoke when, what was said etc. Remember to treat every stage as 'strange'. Use the photograph on page 21 to help you.**

Points to note about 'applied' phenomenology are:

- only small scale studies are done (eg one ward in a hospital);
- no 'laws' or general statements about social behaviour are made, only descriptions of behaviour and suggestions about the underlying common sense ideas of the participants;
- the researcher must make great effort at every moment of the study not to take *anything* for granted.

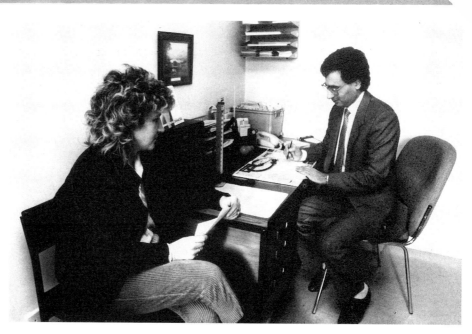

'Consulting the doctor'—see exercise opposite.

☐ **1 Why are the studies small scale, and why do they not produce any 'laws' of social behaviour?**

2 What other areas concerned with health, welfare and poverty might be suitable for this sort of study?

3 Are there any ways in which this approach could be useful to social policy makers?

4 Have you any general criticisms of the phenomenological perspective and ethnomethodology?

Interactionism

Interactionism concentrates on interpersonal behaviour in small groups, particularly on the effect the attitudes and beliefs held by one person or group can have on another's behaviour and perception. It is based on the following assumptions:

● that perception of ourselves and others is based on symbols or labels (eg I am shy, you are moody and unpredictable, she is intelligent and knowledgeable, he is unreliable, they are stupid, lazy and prone to crime);
● these labels are not necessarily based on fact;
● however they influence our behaviour and that of others;
● and actions based on them can make the image become reality;
● though equally people may reject labels, dispel them and create new ones.

Thus the labels or images we have of other people and groups (and of ourselves) are in a constant state of flux, of negotiation and renegotiation. Some are more durable than others, and some are only partial. When we meet someone new we have the elements of a label ready for them (because of the way they speak and look, the clothes they are wearing, the way they behave and so on). We merely need to fill in the details. All of these things will be influenced by that person's self-perception and the image they are trying to create. Having fixed an idea of 'what this person is like', we behave towards them in a particular way and this will influence the way they behave with us. Meanwhile, of course, the same process is occurring for the other person. We do not even have to meet people for this process to occur—images are formed about black people, football supporters and drug takers, for example, from all sorts of sources. These images may influence our behaviour in many ways.

T. Robinson, in *In Worlds Apart: Professionals and their Clients in the Welfare State*, notes how the symbols of the medical profession are used by doctors to control the situation. This starts from the moment the patient enters the room:

> 'she is faced by a white-coated doctor often behind his desk, sometimes surrounded by some of the esoteric symbols of his profession. He may well also have a deferential bevy of medical students, an odd nurse and maybe a visitor or two ... In that situation the consultant clearly controls the whole encounter. Everyone waits on his questions, actions and movements. Frequently he will ask questions of the [patient] with little explanation of their relevance and will make little attempt to explain what he makes of the answers. Taken *in toto* a very powerful message of the importance ... and strange expertise of the doctor is spelt out and the [patient] who feels sufficiently at home, confident and significant to take an active part in what is going on is probably the exception'. (p 39)

Other sociologists have noted the consequences of this sort of interaction for various groups. Ann Cartwright has found that the working class receive inferior treatment from the medical profession because, being labelled as uneducated and unlikely to understand explanations given to them, they are rarely given such explanations (see page 66). Erving Goffman documents the consequences of interactions in mental institutions (page 89) and Ann Oakley and Hilary Graham show how pregnancy and childbirth are perceived in very different ways by doctors and mothers, with the doctor's approach prevailing (see page 82).

☐ In what areas of the fields of health, welfare and poverty are these insights relevant?

☐ 1 In what ways could policy makers implement the insights offered by this perspective?

2 Are studies based on an interactionist perspective necessarily small scale like those of phenomenology?

3 What criticisms have you of the interactionist perspective?

The New Right

The New Right philosophy appears to be the dominant one in the western world today. Mrs Thatcher and President Bush subscribe to it. Even Mr Gorbachev has tried to implement some of its teachings in the USSR.

The New Right (also known as neo-conservatives, market liberals and anti-collectivists) are developing the thought of the 'old right'—most notably Adam Smith, the political economist. Both the new and the old right believe that:

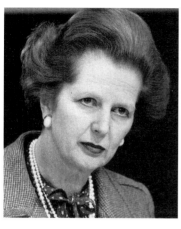

Mrs Thatcher, leader of the New Right in Britain.

● the capitalist system is capable of providing wealth and happiness for all,
● through the operation of the market system, which ensures that prices and wages find their correct level so that there is full employment and a match between supply and demand,
● however governments mistakenly try to interfere in the market through taxation, welfare measures and artificial restrictions on companies' activities,
● which leads to wages that are too high (and so to expensive goods that cannot be sold abroad), unemployment (because of high wages and the attractions of welfare benefits) and lack of initiative (because high taxation means there is no reward for risk-taking).

Some of the strongest proponents of this anti-government philosophy have senior posts in Conservative governments. Not least of these is Margaret Thatcher.

Their specific arguments against the welfare state are summarised on page 13. They do not suggest that the welfare state should be abolished, however, merely that welfare policy should be in line with the 'residual model'—ie those who need state help form a small group at the bottom of society. Benefits should be targeted at them (and only them) and should be minimal. Universal provision of benefits is nonsensical; it gives to those who don't need it and wastes resources. Child Benefit, for example, costs nearly £5 billion a year (1988), going to 6·8 million households with 12 million children regardless of income.

The vertical and static nature of the residual model

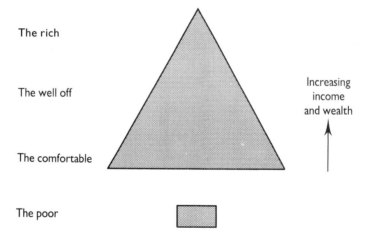

The residual model relies on the ability of the caring agencies to identify those in need. This is done primarily through the use of means testing. Benefits can thus be targeted to those who need them. Means tested welfare is cheap, efficient and effective. Its effectiveness is a double one in that, being cheap, taxes can be reduced and the incentive to work is increased as a result. This will increase the prosperity of the country in the long term. Also, means testing limits demands for goods and services. For example, charging for eye tests and dental check ups (free prior to 1989) will cut any unnecessary demands for these services.

☐ **What arguments are there *against* means testing and in *favour* of universal benefits?**

☐ **What five policies would have priority for implementation if you headed a newly-elected government with a strong New Right philosophy?**

What criticisms have you of the New Right perspective?

The 1986 Social Security Act, summarised on page 15, reflected the Conservative's New Right philosophy in the following ways:

- by emphasising the family (eg by denying benefit to young people who, without a job, leave their families);
- by attempting to encourage self-reliance and independence (for example by encouraging people to take care of their own pensions and by making people pay back money borrowed from the Social Fund);
- in its residual model of welfare, giving only to the worst off (for example by making the Social Fund a last resort).

Social Democrats

Social Democrats base their views on the twin pillars of J. M. Keynes and W. Beveridge. Keynes provided the economic theory, Beveridge the social component of their thought. Keynes argued that the government could manage demand for goods and employment levels in the economy through careful intervention, eg by its own spending and taxing policies. Beveridge argued in favour of compulsory insurance for each member of society to protect them against the hazards of a market economy. *Everybody* should be insured and *everybody* should be eligible to receive state benefits. This '*institutional* model' of welfare contrasts strongly with the New Right's residual model, which, in the eyes of Social Democrats, leads to social division and the marginalisation of the poor and needy. Beveridge believed that it was the duty of the individuals in society to stand together, the strong supporting the weak. Though for some it may mean that the costs of welfare were more than the benefits received, they at least had the satisfaction of contributing to the general good and knowing that if they should fall on hard times they too would be supported by the community.

The horizontal and dynamic nature of the institutional model

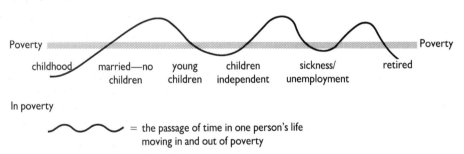

Out of poverty

Poverty ▓▓▓▓▓▓▓▓▓▓▓▓▓▓▓▓▓▓▓▓▓▓▓▓▓▓ Poverty

childhood   married—no children   young children   children independent   sickness/ unemployment   retired

In poverty

〜〜〜 = the passage of time in one person's life moving in and out of poverty

The advantages of a unified system of social insurance over separate policies administered by private companies were claimed by Beveridge to be:

- convenience—only one authority to deal with
- no demarcation problems—ie disputes between bodies about responsibility
- no gaps in cover
- absolute security of benefit

□ **Sweden is often seen as the social-democratic ideal. Find out as much as you can about the welfare system in Sweden and prepare a presentation about it for the group you are studying with. (R. Mishra's book *The Welfare State in Crisis* may be of help.)**

□ **List three social institutions *other than* the church and the family. What functions do they perform for society?**

- uniform rates and conditions
- uniformity of procedure
- economies in administrative costs through concentration of administration in one body.

Functionalism

Functionalism is a sociological perspective which sees social organisation as possessing many similarities to the physical make-up of an animal's body. Both the body and society consist of distinguishable parts (legs, eyes etc for the one, the church, family etc for the other). In both animals and society the parts all play some clear role, ie they fulfil a function, (movement, sight etc, social integration, human reproduction etc). In both, too, the different parts act together to form a system which (usually) operates smoothly to fulfil the goals of the whole. The functionalists maintain, then, that:

- societies are made up of social institutions (the parts)
- which perform identifiable functions
- and together make up the social system (the interacting whole).

So functionalism, at least in its early days (the end of the last century and the first half of this one), tended to see everything which existed in society as fulfilling some sort of function. As in animals, there was no room for dead-weight—anything which was not of use was eliminated by natural selection.

Functionalism as applied to the study of health, welfare and poverty makes the following assertions:

- That poverty is functional for society: it motivates people to do menial jobs, creates jobs in the 'caring' professions, makes those not in poverty feel good, provides incentives for social mobility and so on.
- However, those marginalised by excessive poverty may cause social upheaval by civil unrest, even revolution.
- The institutions of the Welfare State are therefore necessary to integrate the marginalised into society through putting a limit on the deprivation they suffer. Both poverty (at a certain level) and the Welfare State (appropriately developed) are useful to society.

The functionalist view on ill health was elaborated by one of the best known functionalists, Talcott Parsons. He studied psychology in the early part of his career, and perhaps as a result concluded that most ill-health was psycho-somatic (ie the result of pyschological rather than physical factors). Often, becoming ill is the result of a conscious or unconscious *decision* by people, usually because their normal role obligations in society have become too demanding. Exposure to infection or accident can occur in this way. Minor ailments may be imagined to be serious and may even become so because of the response of the patient. Mental illness can also be the result of such choices by the individual, in Parson's view.

By becoming 'ill' the patient is escaping into a sick-role. This has four main aspects according to Parsons. They are:

- the sick person is exempt from certain social responsibilities

- s/he cannot be expected to take care of him/herself or get rid of the illness by 'willpower'
- s/he should want to be well
- s/he should seek medical advice and cooperate with medical experts.

The sick role is functional in that it prevents the formation of a subculture of the sick. Such a subculture would be disruptive to the social system as it would develop a set of norms and values which legitimated incapacity, fatalism, dependency, non-work and so on. The sick-role prevents this by ensuring that the sick person interacts with doctors, friends and relatives, not other sick people. The sick-role also denies legitimacy to being sick because of the final two points outlined above. Thus, it helps avoid the situation in which a significant number of the population become sick in order to avoid work and other social responsibilities.

Table 1: Parson's analysis of the roles of patients and doctors

Patient: sick role	Doctor: professional role
Obligations and Privileges 1. Must want to get well as quickly as possible 2. Should seek professional medical advice and cooperate with the doctor 3. Allowed (and may be expected) to shed some normal activities and responsibilities (eg employment, household tasks) 4. Regarded as being in need of care and unable to get better by his or her own decision and will	*Expected to* 1. Apply a high degree of skill and knowledge to the problems of illness 2. Act for welfare of patient and community rather than for own self-interest, desire for money, advancement, etc 3. Be objective and emotionally detached (ie should not judge patients' behaviour in terms of personal value system or become emotionally involved with them) 4. Be guided by rules of professional practice *Rights* 1. Granted right to examine patients physically and to enquire into intimate areas of physical and personal life 2. Granted considerable autonomy in professional practice 3. Occupies position of authority in relation to the patient

Source: D. L. Patrick and G. Scambler, *Sociology as applied to Medicine* Balliere Tindall, 1986.

To sum up, then, the functionalist position on health, welfare and poverty is that:

- the institutions concerned with these issues (the Welfare State, poverty, the sick role) are functional,
- in that they keep society integrated and working properly,
- but that it is important that the levels of poverty, ill-health and so on are neither too high nor too low.
- Thus the welfare aspects of the social system need constantly to monitor and adapt to the changing levels to ensure balance (a process of 'homoeostasis'—stability through movement).

☐ 1 **In what ways could policy makers implement the insights offered by this perspective?**

2 **Are studies based on a functionalist perspective likely to be small scale or large scale? Why?**

3 **What criticisms have you of the functionalist perspective?**

Functionalists differ from Marxists, whom we will examine next, in that while functionalists see society as based on agreement and operating in the interests of all, Marxists see it as based on exploitation and conflict. However there are similarities; both see the demands of the whole social system as determining the development of welfare institutions within it. Both see individuals as relatively unimportant; they are merely part of larger social institutions (the economic system, classes). Both see these institutions as operating in a functional manner, though for the Marxists the functions are being performed for the benefit of only a few people in society rather than for all.

Marxism

Marxism sees societies which have existed so far as being divided into two (though sometimes more) social classes which have directly competing interests. In the British system, capitalism, the workers— who are trying to sell their labour for the highest price—are in direct competition, and sometimes conflict, with the capitalists—who are trying to cut costs and maximise profits by paying the lowest possible wages.

Preparing the next generation of the proletariat?

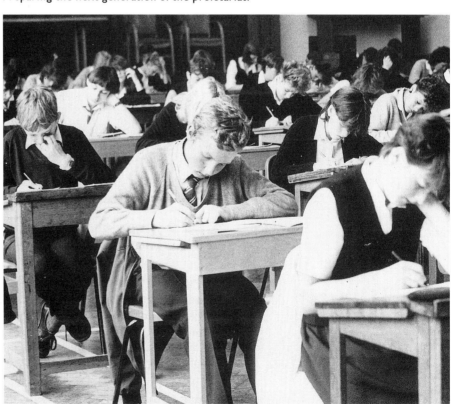

The main elements of the Marxist view of the Welfare State are as follows:

- the Welfare State was created to pacify the working class by giving them a stake in society and (through the discipline imposed by the education system) making them obedient to their employers.
- Actually it benefits the capitalists most by giving them a healthy, well-housed, state-subsidised and well educated workforce with a reserve army of labour, maintained by the DSS, ready if required.
- The costs for this are borne not by the capitalists but by the state with money raised through a taxation system. The tax burden falls most heavily on those who can least afford it.
- The Welfare State was never designed to eradicate poverty or reduce social inequality—its main principle is merely to ensure that no-one starves, thus reducing the chances of a violent revolution.
- The rich benefit from the Welfare State not only because it provides them with a suitable workforce, but because it also gives them benefits through the tax system (relief on mortgages, company cars and expense accounts etc) as well as direct benefits (such as free or subsidised schooling, higher education, health care, transport and so on).

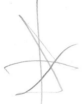

Some Marxists have a rather more positive view of the Welfare State. For example, for Gough the growth of social expenditure in the 1960s and 70s was the product of working class pressure on the state. As there was then full employment, unions could use the threat of strikes to push for more concessions both from employers and the state. Indeed, Marx himself believed nineteenth century welfare measures were implemented under pressure of working class action.

Marxists have a distinctive view of biomedicine as well as the Welfare State. For them, capitalist medicine is used as a means of social control, manipulating behaviour to keep it within the bounds of the 'normal'. Some of the ways this is done are:

- alleviating the symptoms caused by an unhealthy capitalist system, thus making that system more bearable (treating the headache, not the noisy working conditions that caused it);
- legitimating official attempts to change people's behaviour by deeming that behaviour to be both unhealthy and indulged in only by weak or stupid people (advising against promiscuity, illegal drug use, etc);
- acting as a gate-keeper, by ensuring that only those who are 'acceptably sick' are allowed to have time away from work with pay.

There are many similarities between the apparently opposed perspectives of the New Right and Marxism. They agree that everyone wants the government to spend more, but doesn't want higher taxes. They agree that there is government overload so that its job is not done effectively, and there are insufficient resources. They agree that welfare benefits and services often go to people who don't need them.

There are similarities, too, with the functionalists. Marxists like O'Connor are really arguing that the Welfare State is functional for the capitalist economic and social system. The functionalists would not disagree with this (though they would use different terms). More recent

☐ **Has Marxism anything useful to say to policy makers? What criticisms have you of the Marxist perspective?**

Marxists have, however, moved away from this 'functionalist Marxism', particularly in seeking to show the contradictions between a capitalist state and a welfare state (especially the 'fiscal crisis' or what A. Gunder-Frank calls 'welfare farewell').

Feminism

Feminism sees the welfare system as incorporating the patriarchal (male-dominated) ideology found in the rest of society. Examples to illustrate this are numerous, but some of the best-known ones are as follows:

- The insurance system which existed between the two world wars largely excluded married women—they were considered to be the responsibility of their husbands.
- The family-household system is a miniature welfare system which relies on the unpaid and unrecognised work of women.
- Prior to the European Court finding the rule discriminatory in the mid 1980s, married women could not claim Attendance Allowance for looking after a disabled relative (caring was their responsibility anyway, the thinking ran), though men (married or single) and single women could.
- Married men and men cohabiting with a woman claim benefit for both where both are eligible, the female cannot claim in her own right.
- Women are expected to take the burden of welfare from the state by looking after elderly and sick relatives, especially with the advent of 'community care' (see page 102).
- Women bear the brunt of poor housing and low levels of benefit, as men give them the responsibility for staying at home, feeding the family and so on.
- Until very recently married women's income tax affairs had to be handled by their husbands so that the woman was legally obliged to disclose all her financial information to the man, but not vice versa.
- The education system has traditionally given restricted access to females and continues to serve them badly.

As far as poverty is concerned, many of those who are in poverty are women. This is because:

- women tend to be found in low-paid, part-time and insecure jobs;
- women live longer and are therefore disproportionately found among the elderly poor;
- as women are deemed responsible for child-care, they are likely to have gaps in payments into penson funds and National Insurance which mean lower benefits on retirement.

Women's health is discussed extensively in Chapter 5. Here we need merely note that women suffer worse physical and mental health than men.

The root causes of this situation are interpreted differently by different schools of feminism. For Marxist feminists the above facts result from women's role in servicing the capitalist system. By having and caring for children they reproduce the proletariat for capitalists, at

☐ Feminists identify a number of problems in the fields of health, welfare and poverty. In groups, describe six social changes you would recommend to put these problems right. Then compare your lists.

What criticisms have you of the feminist perspective?

☐ If you are studying in a group, divide yourselves into seven small groups and each one select one of the perspectives outlined in this chapter. Prepare to conduct a discussion on one of the following issues:

● The future of the NHS;
● The role of the family in health, welfare and poverty;
● The causes of poverty.

the same time as keeping the current generation well-fed, housed and happy. All this at no cost to the capitalists. The family-household system is the principle method by which this is achieved, so Marxist feminists wish to abolish this as well as making fundamental changes to the economic system.

Radical feminists identify men in general rather than the male capitalists in particular as responsible for women's oppression. For many of them the answer lies in withdrawal from and opposition to the patriarchal society and its welfare institutions. Women's self-help groups, hospitals and clinics for women only, women's cooperatives and so on, offer the best chance for escaping from the situation.

For the more 'moderate' liberal feminists, there is nothing immutable about the current situation. Reform is possible and women can implement changes by getting into positions of power from which they can make changes. Public opinion can be changed through the media and through pressure group activity. Sexist laws can be repealed (as in the example of Attendance Allowance and income tax law above) and new legislation (such as the Sex Discrimination Act) brought in.

Document A

'A state which does for its citizens what they can do for themselves is an evil state ... In such an irresponsible society no-one cares, no-one saves, no-one bothers—why should they when the state spends all its energies taking money from the energetic, successful and thrifty to give to the idle, the failures and the feckless?'

Document B

'After trial of a different principle, it has been found to accord best with the sentiments of the British people that in insurance organised by the community by use of compulsory powers each individual should stand in on the same terms; none should claim to pay less because he is healthier or has more regular employment. In accord with that view, the proposals of the report mark another step forward to the development of State insurance as a new type of human institution, differing both from the former methods of preventing or alleviating distress and from voluntary insurance. The term 'social insurance' to describe this institution implies both that it is compulsory and that men stand together with their fellows. The term implies a pooling of risks ...'

■ a) Identify which perspective these two quotes come from.
   b) What reasons are there for your answer?
   c) Choose one *other* perspective on health, welfare and poverty and show how it would react to the ideas expressed in documents A and B.

☐ Though these have all been called 'perspectives' it may be more precise to say that some are *political ideologies* while others are *sociological perspectives*. Listed below are the characteristic features of both of these. After reading about each perspective, and using any other knowledge you may have about it, tick the appropriate boxes under the statements. Sociological perspectives should have 5 ticks in the left column, political ideologies 5 in the right column (the boxes represent the perspectives, with the initial above each).

Sociological perspective		**Political ideology**
1. Describes how society works	**OR**	Makes judgements about the 'good' society
P ☐ I ☐ NR ☐ SD ☐ FNC ☐ M ☐ FMNSM ☐		P ☐ I ☐ NR ☐ SD ☐ FNC ☐ M ☐ FMNSM ☐
2. Is interested in all facets of the operation of society	**OR**	Tends to concentrate on certain parts of society's operation, particularly on how resources are (or should be) distributed to individuals and groups within society
P ☐ I ☐ NR ☐ SD ☐ FNC ☐ M ☐ FMNSM ☐		P ☐ I ☐ NR ☐ SD ☐ FNC ☐ M ☐ FMNSM ☐
3. Is based on a well-developed theory	**OR**	Is based on values
P ☐ I ☐ NR ☐ SD ☐ FNC ☐ M ☐ FMNSM ☐		P ☐ I ☐ NR ☐ SD ☐ FNC ☐ M ☐ FMNSM ☐
4. Has a body of knowledge, based on research, to support it	**OR**	Uses any available evidence that supports its case
P ☐ I ☐ NR ☐ SD ☐ FNC ☐ M ☐ FMNSM ☐		P ☐ I ☐ NR ☐ SD ☐ FNC ☐ M ☐ FMNSM ☐
5. Suggests strategies for the successful study of society	**OR**	Suggests policies for the improvement of society
P ☐ I ☐ NR ☐ SD ☐ FNC ☐ M ☐ FMNSM ☐		P ☐ I ☐ NR ☐ SD ☐ FNC ☐ M ☐ FMNSM ☐

☐ **Construct a matrix with seven sections along the vertical axis (one for each of the perspectives we have examined) and eight along the horizontal axis. This gives 56 boxes. Along the top of the matrix put the following questions, in turn, above each section.**

Does it focus on interpersonal behaviour?
Does it take a national perspective?
Does it favour major change in the welfare system?
Does the Welfare State significantly alter the social structure?
Does it prefer a quantitative or qualitative methodology?
Who benefits most from the Welfare State?
Who loses most from the Welfare State?
Are there any 'baddies'?

Now, either alone or taking one perspective each (alone or in small groups), complete the boxes.

☐ **1 Which perspectives do the following statements illustrate?**

'The state can do most for the poor by encouraging them to help themselves.'
'United action to change the institutions which make them poor is the only long-term solution to poverty. It must be done by the poor themselves.'
'The state has a responsibility towards the sick, poor and helpless.'

Write three similar statements to illustrate different perspectives.

2 Individually, finish the following sentences as they would be finished by someone subscribing to the perspective in brackets after them:

'Because the decision-makers are all men ...' (Feminist)

'By studying the doctor–patient relationship ...'
(interactionist)
'In an egalitarian society ...' (functionalist)
'The point of treating a situation as "strange" is ...'
(phenomenologist)

Write a similar list of five 'starts' and hand them to your fellow students to finish.

☐ If you are studying in a large group, divide into five smaller groups and choose one of the following roles.

The New Right
The Marxists
The Social Democrats
The Functionalists
The Feminists

Each should:

a) come up with a set of welfare policies on the 'five giants':
education
health
unemployment
housing
poverty.

b) explain why it thinks the old-style welfare policies (1946–1979) were in need of change, and particularly why they failed to eliminate each of the five giants. Explain also how your group's new policies will work to eliminate those giants.

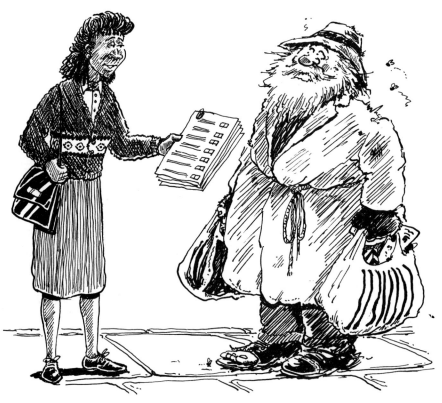

Just complete this and post it back to me at the University, would you?

☐ **What would a better method of study be here?**

Asking questions

☐ **Perspectives, such as those discussed earlier, and the methods outlined in this table, are linked, in that some perspectives are more likely to use particular sorts of methods than others. Which of these methods do you think would be suited to each perspective, and why?**

Table 2 The methods of research available to the student of health, welfare and poverty

More quantitative	More qualitative
PRIMARY DATA (collected by the researcher) this includes ...	
Asking questions	
structured interviews closed-ended questionnaires (ie tick-the-box answers)	unstructured interviews open-ended questionnaires life histories group discussions
Observation	
non-participant observation (can be quantitative or qualitative)	participant observation
Experiments	
controlled experiments (in the laboratory —including animal studies)	uncontrolled experiments (in real situations outside the laboratory)
SECONDARY DATA (obtained from other sources)	
official statistics	diaries, letters, auto-biographies etc.

Questionnaires

Closed-ended

'Heartbeat Wales', a government-backed health education pilot project, has spent two years analysing a survey of Welsh families which asked people aged between 12 and 64 detailed questions on their attitudes to health, their medical history and use of health services. In total, 22,000 people were covered, the largest survey of its kind in Britain.

Open-ended

For *Poverty in the United Kingdom* Peter Townsend used a questionnaire which combined both open and closed-ended questions about households. The major survey work was conducted between 1968–9 in 51 constituencies in the UK. Follow-up surveys were conducted later in Salford, Neath, Glasgow and Belfast. In total, data on 2,052 households (6,098 individuals) was successfully collected in the main survey. Examples of open-ended questions include 'If there is poverty, what do you think can be done about it?', and 'What kinds of things have you done lately to try to get a job?'

Interviews

Structured

The Government's Health and Life-Style Survey uses in-depth interview techniques combined with measurements of blood-pressure, lung-

☐ **Try writing structured questions designed to elicit this information. Swap yours with other members of the group for constructive criticism.**

function etc. It aims to establish correlations between the nature of individuals' health and life-style and their income, social class, education and housing. Questions include ones on self-perceived health, ability to sleep well and so on.

Unstructured

In *Poverty: The Forgotten Englishmen*, Coates and Silburn describe a study which they organised of poverty in the St Ann's district of Nottingham. The team conducted interviews in three stages, the first with a sample of nearly 200, the second of under 100 and the third over 200. The research was conducted between 1966 and 1968. Few details of the interview schedule are given in the book, but it's clear from quotes of the responses that it was at least partly unstructured. One old lady, on being asked to describe her financial situation said she was 'not wealthy at all, but I just about get by. Of course, my boys are very good' (p 60). People in the sample were also asked what 'wealth' was. They were allowed to answer as they wanted.

Life histories

☐ **What are the strengths and weaknesses of the 'life history' approach?**

R. Sherrott interviewed 50 people who were volunteers for various sorts of charitable and other work. He took life histories from each of them, encouraging them to speak frankly about their current and past involvement in voluntary work, their social situation, and their feelings and experiences. The result has been described as 'a rich portrait of volunteering'. Sherrott found that there were many motives for volunteering, from instrumental reasons (for example to enhance employment prospects) to normative ones (the belief in the need for a strong community) to moral ones (volunteering as a means of doing one's duty to God or society).

Group discussions

B. Mostyn also conducted a study of volunteering, first using group discussions, and later with semi-structured interviews. For the first, houses were selected at random in a particular area, the people inside were told about the study, given a questionnaire about their involvement in voluntary work and, if they qualified to join in terms of their class and age (a mixed group of participants being required), asked if they would be willing to take part in a group discussion on volunteeering. These were held in community halls hired for the occasion. There were a total of six separate discussion groups, three in York and three in London. A total of 46 people attended. She found that most respondents agreed on the following hierarchy of status in voluntary agencies and volunteering:

Altruistic volunteering, eg Samaritans, Mountain Rescue, St John's Ambulance
Helping people in distress, eg Salvation Army, fostering
Giving aid to the less fortunate, eg Citizens Advice Bureau, Friends of the Hospital, Round Table
Improving society, eg Youth leaders, school governors, Residents' Associations
Self interest, eg Trade Union work, Party activists, local pressure groups

Townsend's questionnaire

QUESTION 14   Fuel

Everyone forgets to order coal. Stress "through lack of money".

QUESTION 15   Birthday parties

Again the emphasis is on the expense and the experience of bringing the child's friends into the home, so stress that we don't mean just a family party.

QUESTION 17 (a)   Social class

This question requires the views of both chief wage-earner (head of household) and housewife. By "chief wage-earner" we mean the person upon whose earnings the housekeeping income primarily depends. By "Head of Household" we have in mind the alternative person to be questioned if there is no chief wage-earner, e.g. a husband who is a retirement pensioner, or a widowed mother (who may be the tenant) living with her widowed daughter (the housewife) and grandchildren. As far as possible the views on social class should be sought from each person independently. If both are present take the question stage by stage, making sure both answer before passing on. The question asks first for a self-rating, which must be written down. At this stage avoid putting names of classes into people's heads. People often hesitate awkwardly, so try to get the informant to say what class she thinks she belongs to or "is nearest to". Prompt by repeating the question carefully, and say "It's what you think", implying (which is true) that everyone has their own idea and each is equally valid. Do not strain to get an answer if one is not easily forthcoming. Do not assume the informant will pick one class only. Multiple choices of "middle and working" or "professional and working" are allowed.

QUESTION 17 (b)   Determinant of class

Code housewife and chief wage-earner only. Next, to give us a clue as to what the informant is using as a reference point and scale we ask, in effect, the informant's idea of what determines "class". Try to get the most important one only.

QUESTION 17 (c)   Names of classes

Third, the informant is presented with a flash-card (this is why husband and wife should if possible be interviewed separately, since otherwise the second person may be unduly influenced). Code one item only. If informant wants (again) to say "None", say 'Well, I've got to put something down, which would you think was nearest?" This rating is the most important bit of the question. Do not be puzzled if the wife gives a different answer from the husband. This is quite common.

QUESTION 17 (d)   Father's main occupation

That is, the occupation held for most of the time (not necessarily the most recent).

QUESTION 18   Well off

Four comparisons are made in this series of questions—with relatives, with other people (note—of the same age) in locality, with the average in the country and finally in the context of time. Prompt carefully and remember that you might get a different response for one comparison than for another.

Source: P. Townsend, *Poverty in the United Kingdom*, Penguin

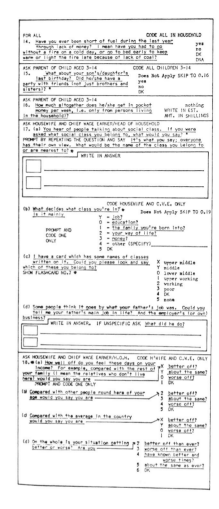

☐ **Townsend's questionnaire was administered by researchers. What are the advantages and disadvantages of this approach compared to, say, sending it through the post?**

Observation

Participant observation

The authors of the book *A Cycle of Deprivation?* decided that participant observation of four 'deprived' families was the best way to understand the nature and causes of their deprivation. Accordingly, they studied four carefully chosen families in 'Kindleton' (somewhere in the English Midlands) over a period of two years in the mid 1970s:

> 'We were temporary participant-observers entering the lives of our families, sometimes for a short visit and on other occasions for a whole day; at times we just talked to members of the families and at other times joined a birthday party, a family christening or other family celebrations'. (page 12)

Their finding was that the concept of a 'cycle of deprivation' (see page 50 for an explanation of this) is too simple a concept to explain the lives of the four families they studied. A 'web' of deprivation is a more adequate metaphor. The authors wish to stress the complexity of the families' situation and the fact that the multiple deprivations they suffer are interacting and cumulative.

> 'We would claim that no single hypothesis and no group of simple hypotheses could hope to explain the intricate mesh of factors which we have listed when summarizing the crucial features of any one family at the end of each chapter.' (p 163)

□ 1 **What are:**
   a) **the advantages**
   b) **the disadvantages**
   of the choice of participant observation as the research method for this study?

2 **Given that a non-sociologist such as George Orwell can use this method in his book *Down and Out In Paris and London*, and that the results of the method read more like newspaper journalism than a scientific account, is there any point in studying sociology if participant observation is the method you decide to use?**

3 **Participant observation can be overt or covert. Under what circumstances would covert participant observation be advisable and why?**

Non-participant observation

The earliest studies of poverty tended to use NPO in assessing its nature and extent. Charles Booth's *Life and Labour of the People in London* is an example of the indirect use of NPO. Booth met the London School Board visitors responsible for the East End, the area he was interested in. These officials visited homes in the area and they kept very detailed written accounts of every family with children of school age or pre-school age there. Thus Booth was able to gain a clear picture of conditions at the end of the nineteenth century using NPO by a team of trained and skilled workers.

□ **What are the advantages and disadvantages of Booth's approach?**

Experiments

Controlled

These attempt to keep all important conditions constant, and usually have two identical groups for testing; the *experimental* and, for comparison, the *control*. One variable is introduced or changed in the experimental group, but not the control. Any subsequent differences between the two should therefore be the result of that variable. In tests of the effectiveness of a medicine, the medicine is administered to the experimental group. The control group, who are usually matched in terms of age, health etc, get a placebo—some 'treatment' which is known to be ineffective. The point in doing this is that receiving treatment of *any* kind can sometimes have an effect on the patient. Administering a placebo means both are receiving some treatment. It is best if the experiment is a 'double blind' one, ie neither those conducting the experiment nor those being experimented on know who is receiving the medicine and who the placebo.

Controlled experiments have taken place to test the effectiveness of alternative medicine. One was a test of acupuncture's ability to control disabling breathlessness. Twelve matched pairs of patients with this problem were selected. One of each of the pairs was given acupuncture treatment, the other placebo acupuncture (ie what appeared to be acupuncture but was not). After three weeks' treatment those people who had received acupuncture felt significantly greater benefit than those having the placebo.

Experiments on young animals have been done to test the effect of malnutrition on brain growth. Control and experimental animals were kept in laboratory conditions, the latter being deprived of adequate food for long periods of time. Later analysis of the brains of both sets of animals showed that the experimental group had fewer and smaller brain cells than is normal. It seems that malnutrition during the period of most rapid brain growth (the first six months after birth) can irrevocably result in this deficiency.

□ **What factors make controlled experiments in sociology more difficult and unreliable than those in the natural sciences?**

Uncontrolled field experiment

This sort of experiment is uncontrolled in the sense that not all conditions are kept constant. The experimental and control groups are not identical, neither are the conditions in which they exist. One study in the Birmingham area looked at a sample of boys between six and seven and another between ten and 11. Some of the boys were from severely deprived large families known to the social services department. The rest (the control group) lived in the same area but were not under social services supervision. Differences such as height, visual impairment, hearing loss, disease and so on were examined. It was found that the experimental group (known to social services) tended to be shorter, more often ill and to suffer worse vision and hearing than those not known to social services.

Secondary data

Statistics

We can infer the levels of health and illness from official statistics. There are four categories of these:

- mortality statistics—eg the infant mortality rate (IMR);
- statistics on the use of health facilities (eg the Hospital In-Patient Enquiry—HIPE) or studies of GP's case loads;
- statistics on sickness absence from work;
- statistics collected from official surveys. These include the General Household Survey, an annual survey of a representative sample of people in Britain, and The National Food Survey—a questionnaire sent annually to a sample of the population by the Ministry of Agriculture.

The Office of Population Censuses and Surveys' longitudinal study uses a combination of statistical sources. It has followed vital events in the lives of a sample of 1% of the population of England and Wales since 1971. These include births, marriages, deaths, cancer registrations and so on, all of which can be gleaned from official sources of information such as the census, registrations by doctors, registrars and others, which are all collated by the OPCS.

Each of these categories has its problems:

- Mortality statistics only measure deaths (mortality), not illness (morbidity) and so non-fatal diseases are hidden from view.
- Statistics on the use of health facilities only catch the people who have gone through the process of recognition, definition and action (see page 5).

- Statistics on absence from work because of sickness exclude people not working (for whatever reason), and people who are absent for less than seven days, as short absences do not qualify for sickness benefit and are therefore not recorded.
- Information collected from the General Household Survey tends to underestimate such problems as cancer and mental illness because people are asked about their own health.
- Problems such as a high non-response rate (which particularly affects the National Food Survey), limited sample sizes and difficulties in selecting a truly representative sample mean that there are usually question marks over the statistical significance of results.
- The time taken to collate the results often means that statistics are out of date by the time they become available.
- Political expediency can influence official statistics in many ways. The changing definition of 'the unemployed' is the best known example of how official statistics can be manipulated. For example, after 1982 only those who claimed unemployment benefit were counted as unemployed (as opposed to those registered for work). This change reduced unemployment by 170,000 at a stroke.
- The government can delay the publication of any statistical work it might find embarrassing. It can also limit the number of copies available to the public or try to hush the matter up altogether. This occurred to a study of primary school staff begun in 1987 by the DES and to two surveys on inequalities in health (see page 63).

Despite these problems researchers have been able to use official statistics in their research. Brian Abel-Smith and Peter Townsend in *The Poor and the Poorest* (1965) used figures collected for other purposes by government departments to show that the numbers of those in povery (defined as 40 per cent above the level of National Assistance Benefit) had increased from 4 million in 1953/4 to 7·5 million in 1960, thus casting doubt on the government's assertion to the British people that 'you've never had it so good'.

More generally, the statistics encapsulate medical definitions and diagnoses of ill-health. Each case is different, but doctors have to label each one as they have been trained to do. A death, particularly in old-age, may be the result of many interlinked factors, yet the doctor must state a cause which then becomes a statistic. Moreover, it would hardly be likely that a cause of death such as 'stressful and dangerous work conditions' be entered, though in a sense these could be said to be a 'cause of death'.

☐ **What advantages does using statistics have for the researcher?**

Statistics are useful in that they can enable the researcher to use the comparative method, ie comparison of different countries' statistics to identify the importance of factors which differ between them. Durkheim's use of statistics in studying suicide is a well-known example in Sociology. He claimed to show that societies and communities which have a high level of social integration also have a low level of suicide. So, using statistics, he claimed that too low a level of integration caused a high suicide rate.

☐ **Study Graph A and B, both based on official statistics.**

What do these graphs seem to show?
Why might this be incorrect?

Graph A: Correlation between colon cancer incidence, and meat consumption (1975)

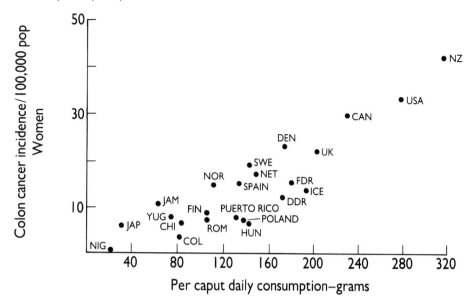

Graph B: Correlation between breast cancer mortality, and fat consumption (1975)

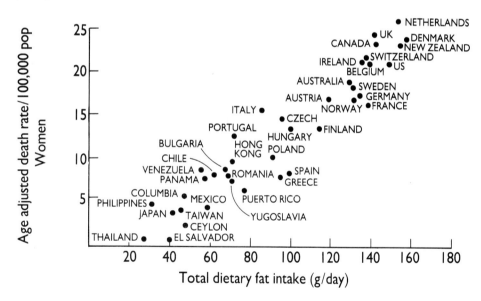

Source: R. Doll and R. Peto, *The Causes of Cancer*, Oxford University Press, 1981

Qualitative secondary data

☐ **Comment on Wilmott's statement and on the titles: *Adolescent Boys of East London* and *Poverty: The Forgotten Englishmen*.**

What are the advantages and disadvantages of Willmott's 'diary method'?

For *Adolescent Boys of East London* P. Willmott asked some of the boys he was studying to keep a week's diary. 30 of them wrote a diary during the same week in 1966 and were given £2 for doing so. Willmott gave them some instructions about the sort of thing he wanted them to write, and an example for them to follow. Later he was able to use this data to describe the lives of the boys. His aim was to examine the processes of male adolescence, especially among the working class. 'Girls', he states, 'pose less of a problem to adult society', as presumably do the middle class.

☐ **Conceptual 20 questions:**

One person in the group chooses a concept from the field of health, welfare and poverty (eg 'the institutional model of welfare'). The rest of the group can ask up to 20 questions—which must be answerable by yes or no—to try to guess what the concept is.

☐ **ESSAY**

Examine the view that the aim of sociology should be to deliver to central government and other policy makers an objective analysis of social problems and clear policy advice about how to solve them.

'I began this book because of a deep commitment to the fundamental principle upon which the NHS was based, that access to health care should not be based upon the ability to pay the costs of treatment, especially during periods of sickness. This was accompanied by a growing anxiety that changes in the private sector since 1979 had undermined that principle. Most of what I have seen and heard in the research for the book has confirmed that view . . .'.

J. Higgins, *The Business of Medicine: Private Health Care in Britain*, Macmillan, London 1988 p 5.

☐ 1 **In what ways, specifically, might the prior values held by researchers influence the course of their research? (Think about the different stages of research; choice of subject, development of a hypothesis, choice of method, analysis of results and so on.) Give examples to illustrate your points.**

2 **How could the research be made as objective as possible, ie so that the results would be the same irrespective of the prior view of the researcher?**

☐ **Which method would be most suitable for studying the following subjects:**

a) **lifestyle and poverty in the gypsy community;**
b) **the relationship between deaths of pensioners during the winter from hypothermia and the levels of state benefits for them;**
c) **the effectiveness of social workers;**
d) **the influence of drug companies' advertising and promotion campaigns on doctors' prescribing habits.**

Bibliography

Blaxter, M. *Evidence on Inequality in Health from a National Survey*, Lancet 1987 ii pp 30–33 (Health and Life-style Survey)

Boyson, R. *Down With the Poor*, in Butterworth, E. and Holman, R. (eds) *Social Welfare in Modern Britain*, Fontana, London 1975 pp. 381–7

Brennan, M. E. *Medical Characteristics of Children Supervised by the Local Authority Social Services Department*, Policy and Politics 1, 1973, 3, p 255

Clarke, J. *et al, Ideologies of Welfare*, Hutchinson, London 1987

Coates, K. and Silburn, R. *Poverty: The Forgotten Englishmen*, Penguin, Harmondsworth 1970

Coffield, F. *et al, A Cycle of Deprivation?*, Heinemann, London 1980

DHSS, *Health and Personal Social Services Statistics for England*, HMSO, London annually

Davis, A. and Horobin, G. (eds), *Medical Encounters: The Experience of Illness and Treatment*, Croom Helm, London 1977

Fried, A. and Elman, M. *Charles Booth's London*, Hutchinson, London 1969

Fry, J., Brooks, D. and McColl, I. *The NHS Data Book*, MTP Press, Lancaster 1984

Gardner, M. J. *et al, Atlas of Mortality from Selected Diseases in England and Wales 1968–1978*, J. Wiley and Sons, Chichester

Gardner, M. J. *et al, Atlas of Cancer Mortality in England and Wales 1968–1978*, J. Wiley and Sons, Chichester

Gough, I. *The Political Economy of the Welfare State*, Macmillan, London 1979

Grant, N. and Middleton, N. *The Daily Telegraph Atlas of the World Today*, Daily Telegraph, London 1984 (see pages 70–71 for IMR)

Hartley, L. *History of Medicine*, Basil Blackwell, Oxford

Hatch, S. *Volunteers: Patterns, Meanings and Motives*, The Volunteer Centre, Berkhamsted 1983

Jordan, B. *Rethinking Welfare*, Basil Blackwell, Oxford 1987

Kane, E. *Doing Your Own Research*, Marion Boyars, London 1984

Kidron, M. and Segal, R. *The State of the World Atlas*, Pluto, London 1984

Kurian, G. T. *The Book of World Ratings*, Macmillan, London 1979

Mishra, R. *Society and Social Policy*, Macmillan, London 1981

O'Connor, J. *The Fiscal Crisis of the State*, Macmillan, London 1981

Office of Health Economics, *Compendium of Health Statistics*, OHE, London 1984 (5th edition)

Open University, *Health and Disease*, U205, see especially *Studying Health and Disease*

Radical Statistics Health Group, *Facing the Figures*, Radical Statistics, London 1987

Robinson, T. in *Worlds Apart: Professionals and their Clients in the Welfare State*, Bedford Square Press, London 1978

Townsend, P. *Poverty in the United Kingdom*, Penguin, Harmondsworth 1979

United Nations, *Statistical Yearbook* and *Demographic Yearbook*, United Nations, New York annually

Willmott, P. *Adolescent Boys of East London*, RKP, London 1966

World Health Organisation, *World Health Statistics Annual Report*, HMSO, London annually

(On page 30, document A is Dr. Rhodes Boyson *Down With the Poor*, and document B is W. Beveridge *Social Insurance and Allied Services*, page 13. The former represents the New Right, the latter the social democrats.)

3 · Poverty

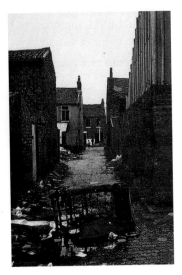

Inner-city Hull in the early 1980s.

What is poverty?

There are three main ways of defining of poverty:

1 Absolute poverty
2 Relative poverty
3 Poverty of lifestyle

Absolute poverty

Early researchers into poverty used this definition. It considers poverty to mean having inadequate income for proper food, clothing and shelter. The most important early studies were Seebohm Rowntree's *Poverty: A Study of Town Life* (published in 1901, a study of York) and Charles Booth's *The Life and Labour of the People of London* (published in 1902 in 17 volumes).

Rowntree's definition of poverty was based on the idea of a measurable subsistence poverty line, below which one did not have the necessities of life. He calculated . . .

'what income is required by families of different sizes to provide the minimum of food, clothing (second hand) and shelter needed for the maintenance of merely physical health.'

If a family fell below this line, then they were poor. In those days 17p was enough to feed one man for a day (10p for a child), though this

☐ Either alone or in groups, describe the circumstances in which someone could be said to be 'in poverty'. Compare your descriptions with others in the group.

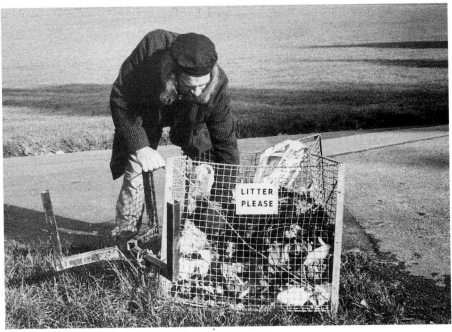

Poverty amid affluence—a tramp on Hampstead Heath, 1980s.

required one to buy from the cheapest shop. To be classified as being in 'primary poverty' a family ...

> 'must never purchase a half penny newspaper or spend a penny to buy a ticket for a popular concert. They must write no letters ... they must never contribute anything to their church or chapel ... the children must have no pocket money ... the father must smoke no tobacco and must drink no beer.'

'Secondary poverty' was the situation in which a family did have enough money to live but some of it was wasted. Rowntree did not necessarily blame the poor for wasting their money. He said their circumstances were often so bad that it was not surprising that they turned to drink or some other expensive habit.

Booth too adopted a harsh definition of poverty, though there are elements of an understanding of relative poverty in his definition (these are italicised):

> 'By the word "poor" I mean ... those who have a sufficiently regular though bare income ... and by "very poor" those who from any cause fall much below this standard. The "poor" are those whose means may be sufficient but are barely sufficient for *decent independent life*, the "very poor" those whose means are insufficient for this *according to the usual standard of life in this country*. My "poor" may be described as living under a struggle to obtain the necessaries of life and make both ends meet, while the "very poor" live in a state of chronic want.'

Relative poverty

K. Galbraith in *The Affluent Society* (1962) said:

> 'People are poverty stricken when their income, even if it is adequate for survival, falls markedly below that of the community. Then they cannot have what the larger community regards as the minimum necessary for decency; and they cannot wholly escape, therefore, the judgement of the larger community that they are indecent. They are degraded for, in the literal sense, they live outside the grades or categories which the community regards as acceptable.'

☐ **List the things that, in Britain, comprise the 'minimum necessary for decency'. If you are working in a group, compare your lists.**

Relative poverty, then, is the state of being poor relative to the community in which one lives. This may result in rejection by the community. It need not necessarily lead to a *feeling* of being poor, though. The subjective experience of deprivation (termed 'relative deprivation' by W. G. Runciman in *Relative Deprivation and Social Justice*) depends on who one compares oneself to—one's 'reference group':

> '... relative deprivation should always be understood to mean a *sense* of deprivation; a person who is "relatively deprived" need not be "objectively" deprived in the more usual sense'.

It is harder to put a precise figure on relative poverty than it is for absolute poverty. Some attempts have been as follows

B. Abel-Smith and P. Townsend, in *The Poor and the Poorest* (1965), used the government's minimum level of benefit and added another 40 per cent. In those days this benefit was called National Assistance Benefit (NAB). It became Supplementary Benefit and then Income Support. In 1986 a family consisting of man, woman and two children (five and ten years old) would be eligible to receive £65·05 plus various other benefits (Housing Benefit, free school meals, prescriptions etc). Abel-Smith and Townsend would consider this to be the *absolute* poverty line. Adding 40 per cent would bring it to a relative poverty line for British society today. This gives a figure of relative poverty for this family of £91·07.

In his more recent *Poverty in the United Kingdom* (1979) Peter Townsend suggested another way of putting a figure on relative poverty. This involves taking the average income and halving it. Thus having an income which is less than half the average person's income would put one in relative poverty.

In 1985 the average gross weekly income for various categories of workers was as follows:

Men (manual)	£163.60
Men (non manual)	£225
Women (manual)	£101.30
Women (non manual)	£133.80
All	£177.00

☐ **What problems are there with the notion that you are in relative poverty if the 'larger community' considers you to be living in an unacceptable way?**

Poverty of lifestyle

This approach to measuring poverty takes into account not just financial factors but also one's whole lifestyle. The idea behind it is that two people may be on the same income (a low one) but only one may have a circle of friends, many interests, plenty of facilities nearby and so on. The other is isolated, perhaps in a depressing inner city environment, with no social contacts and no facilities available. One is in poverty, the other is not. Peter Townsend in *Poverty in the United Kingdom* tried to take such factors into account by giving his sample of respondents a structured interview about their leisure activities and other factors. By an appropriate scoring system he was able to assign an 'index of poverty' to them. Some of the things he asked them about are listed in the table below:

Table 1: Townsend's deprivation index

Characteristic	Percentage of population
1. Has not had a week's holiday away from home in the last 12 months	53.6
2. (Adults only) Has not had a relative or friend to the home for a meal or snack in the last four weeks	33.4
3. (Adults only) Has not been out in the last four weeks to a relative or friend for a meal or snack	45.1
4. (Children under 15 only) Has not had a friend to play or to tea in the last four weeks	36.3
5. (Children only) Did not have a party on last birthday	55.6
6. Has not had an afternoon or evening out for entertainment in the last two weeks	47.0
7. Does not have fresh meat (including meals out) as many as four days a week	19.3

8. Has gone through one or more days in the past fortnight without a cooked meal	7.0
9. Has not had a cooked breakfast most days of the week	67.3
10. Household does not have a refrigerator	45.1
11. Household does not usually have a Sunday joint (three in four times)	25.9
12. Household does not have sole use of four amenities indoors (flush WC; sink or washbasin and cold water tap; fixed bath or shower; and gas or electric cooker)	21.4

Townsend found people on lower incomes tended to have a proportionately high 'index of poverty'. He discovered a threshold of income, below which there was a sudden increase in poverty of lifestyle as measured by the index. This was 1.5 times the Supplementary Benefit level.

One of the main difficulties with this deprivation index is that people may score highly on it not because they are deprived but because they *choose* not to (for example) have a cooked breakfast most days of the week. In a more recent study by Mack and Lansley, there was an attempt to distinguish between styles of living that people could not afford and those they did not choose. One way they did this was by using a questionnaire similar to Townsend's but asking whether they did not have a particular item by choice or because they could not afford it. Also, they tried to establish how far there was agreement between people on what the necessities of life are.

☐ **What problems can you see with this approach to poverty?**

They found that there was a large measure of agreement on this. They used this agreed list of necessities to define poverty; lack of three or more items rendered one 'poor' (though they excluded things like a TV, which very few people lack, and a garden and access to public transport, which will be affected by which part of the country one lives in). Mack and Lansley's results were that 7.5 million people (13.8 per cent of the population) were in poverty in 1983—a lower figure than Townsend's 12.46 million (22.9 per cent) in 1968/9.

☐ **In small teams prepare the following for presentation to the class:**

The Economic and Social Research Council (ESRC) wants a study of poverty conducted in your area. They are offering a grant of £20,000 to do it. The report must be presented in three months' time. You are a team of sociologists and wish to be considered for the project. You therefore have to present a research proposal to the ESRC for their consideration. Your tasks are:

a) **Decide how you will select your sample of people to study.**
b) **Decide on an appropriate definition or definitions of poverty so that you can establish how much of it exists in the area. Give a detailed rationale for your choice and explain why you rejected other alternatives.**
c) **Decide which research method or methods you will use to conduct the research (see Chapter 2). Again, a detailed rationale must be given to the members of the Council.**
d) **Give your research team a name (linked to a university or college?), elect a spokesperson and prepare any visual aids (overhead projector transparencies, photocopied handouts) you need to present your proposal.**

While each group makes its presentation, the others in the class become the members of the ESRC (respected Professors and such). They should try to establish, through questions, which research group to select.

☐ How far does your perception of 'necessities' agree with the general public's? Rank the following list in order of importance, then compare your results with Mack and Lansley's findings (in the bibliography).

Mack and Lansley's jumbled list of necessities

New, not second-hand, clothes	A holiday away from home for one week a year, not with relatives	A roast meat joint or its equivalent once a week
Heating to warm living areas of the home if it's cold	Public transport for one's needs	A 'best outfit' for special occasions
Enough bedrooms for every child over 10 of different sex to have his/her own	A garden	An outing for children once a week
	A television	Meat or fish every other day
Leisure equipment for children, eg sports equipment or a bicycle	A night out once a fortnight (adults)	A dressing gown
	A hobby or leisure activity	Children's friends round for tea/a snack once a fortnight
Carpets in living rooms and bedrooms	Celebrations on special occasions such as Christmas	Indoor toilet (not shared with another household)
Presents for friends or family once a year	Damp-free home	Friends/family round for a meal once a month
Three meals a day for children	A warm water-proof coat	Beds for everyone in the household
	Two hot meals a day (for adults)	Self-contained accommodation
Toys for children	A telephone	A washing machine
Refrigerator	A packet of cigarettes every other day	Two pairs of all-weather shoes
Bath (not shared with another household)		
A car		

Poverty in the UK: the official facts

On 12 July 1988 the Select Committee on Social Services published a report on the extent of poverty in Britain. This was based on official figures and used the lowest level of means-tested benefits as the marker of poverty. The report states that:

- in 1979 4.4 million people were claiming means-tested benefits;
- by 1988 there were 8.2 million;
- in 1988 1 million were below this supposed minimum level.

However, ministers replied that these figures do not demonstrate any increase in poverty in Britain, merely the fact that eligibility for means-tested benefits has relaxed and that levels of benefits have increased. The real measure of poverty should be the poor's spending power, according to ministers. This has increased.

Low-income families

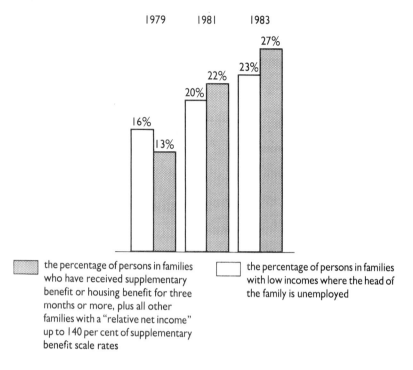

the percentage of persons in families who have received supplementary benefit or housing benefit for three months or more, plus all other families with a "relative net income" up to 140 per cent of supplementary benefit scale rates

the percentage of persons in families with low incomes where the head of the family is unemployed

(a) What trends are revealed here?
(b) What explanations might there be for them?
(c) What dangers are there in using the number of claimants of Supplementary Benefit (now called Income Support) as a measure of poverty in the UK?

Two nations—or three?

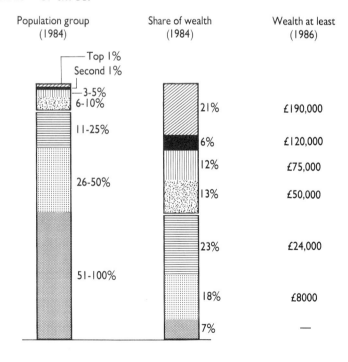

(a) What does this diagram show?
(b) Compare it with the 1985 bar chart on incomes (page 48).

Incomes from 1971 to 1985

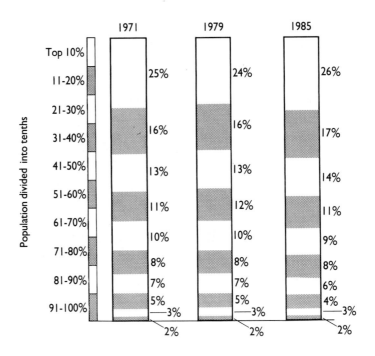

(a) What trends are shown here?
(b) What possible explanations are there for these trends?

The spread of wealth from 1966 to 1984

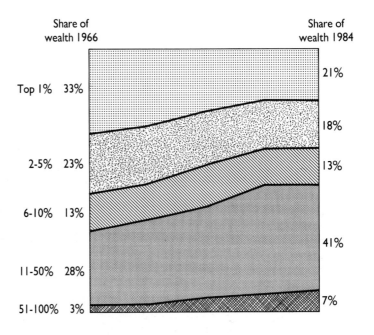

(a) Describe the trends shown here.
**(b) For what reasons might official statistics on
    wealth be inaccurate?**

Source: T. Stark, *The A–Z of Wealth*, tables F, R, C, S, The Fabian Society

Born to succeed? – the status of the millionaires' parents

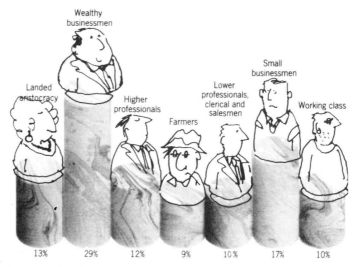

Source : birth certificates of millionaires who died in 1984 or 1985

Source: New Society, 'The Rich in Britain', 22 August 1986

The groups most likely to be poor are:

- the elderly
- single parent families
- the unemployed
- the sick and the disabled
- low wage earners
- those with large families and low incomes.

Explaining poverty

> ☐ **Take each of the four perspectives that follow and show how they might explain the persistence of poverty. If you are working in a large group, divide into smaller groups and take one perspective each. Prepare to explain its view on poverty to the larger group.**

Definitions and explanations of poverty are closely linked to the perspectives we examined earlier. Those which have particularly addressed the issue of poverty are; the New Right, the social democrats, Marxists and functionalists.

The New Right

The New Right adopt an absolute definition of poverty and see it as the fault of the poor people themselves. The poor have a *culture of poverty*. Oscar Lewis argues that people who have a culture of poverty:

- have a low level of literacy and education;
- don't belong to trade unions;
- don't join political parties;
- make little use of banks, hospitals etc;
- are critical of education and the police;
- are poorly organised;
- feel marginalised, helpless and dependent;
- desire immediate gratification rather than deferring it;

□ Do you agree that poor people in Britain have these characteristics? If not, are there any other features which could be said to comprise a 'culture of poverty' in the UK?

□ According to the New Right model:

● Who/what is to blame for the existence of poverty?

● What needs to be done to abolish it?

● Has anything like this been done so far?

● cannot plan for the future;
● are fatalistic (don't believe they can improve the situation);
● believe in male superiority;
● are provincial and have no sense of history.

This attitude to the poor is evident in Mrs Thatcher's talk of the 'dependency culture' which she sees as one of the ills of the Welfare State resulting from over-protectiveness of the 'nanny state'. She wishes to replace it with what she calls the 'enterprise culture'. Similarly former junior health minister Edwina Currie blamed the poor health of those in the North on certain perceived Northern cultural traits, particularly diet and the habit of smoking (and on their ignorance).

Critics of this approach have argued that it blames the victim for the circumstances they are forced to live in. It has also been noted that parents in poverty do not bring their children up in the manner described by culture of poverty theorists. Such parents are usually very keen that their children should have a better life than they had.

Social Democrats

The social democratic approach adopts a relative definition of poverty and accepts the *poverty-trap* (or *cycle of deprivation*) explanation. This suggests that people can get into a situation of poverty and, once there, find it very difficult to get out. Paradoxically it is expensive to be poor and those in poverty have to spend a lot just to maintain their current standard of living. For example:

● the poor cannot afford to insulate their homes and so have to pay high fuel bills;
● they cannot afford to travel to cheap supermarkets out of town and so have to buy goods at the expensive local corner shop;
● they have to buy second-hand cars, washing machines and so on which frequently break down, are expensive to repair and don't give long or continuous service;
● they cannot afford the facilities which allow one to go to work (especially transport and baby minders);
● the welfare benefit system is such that if someone in poverty gets an increase in income (say by getting a better paid job), the benefits they are entitled to are reduced so they end up no better off.

The deprivation cycle

Inadequate parents

Unstable and unsatisfying marriages and family life

Inadequate child-rearing practices

Unskilled job or unemployment, so not enough money to move out of social deprivation

Children deprived emotionally, socially and intellectually

Failure at school

□ Devise other illustrations to demonstrate the viciously circular nature of poverty. Try illustrating the virtuous circle of wealth too.

Source: R. Holman, Poverty: Explanations of Social Deprivation, Martin Robinson, 1978, p 117

In addition to these factors there are longer term 'traps' which mean that the children of those in poverty will also be caught. These include:

- the lack of books in the home which means that poor children are disadvantaged compared to the children of the better off;
- lack of study facilities in small overcrowded homes;
- schools in poor areas tend to be old, lacking in facilities and unpopular with teachers, the best of whom will go elsewhere;
- stereotypes of children from poor homes mean that they are often treated as failures in the first place. As a result they often do fail.

This approach explains why the children of the poor are also disproportionately likely to be poor themselves in later life, despite the fact that their parents may try their best for them. Clearly, this different diagnosis of the causes of inheritance of poverty calls for different treatment.

□ **According to the social democratic model:**

- **Who/what is to blame for the existence of poverty?**
- **What needs to be done to abolish it?**
- **Has anything like this been done so far?**

Marxists

For Marxists, poverty is an inevitable consequence of capitalism. In the capitalist system the wealth of the few is founded upon (and necessitates) the poverty of the many. Marxists very much agree with the old aphorism, 'the rich get richer and the poor get poorer'—the rich are getting richer *because* the poor are getting poorer. The flow of resources from the many to the few works like this, according to Marxists:

- ■ Those in work receive less for their labour than the value they create. This is the source of profit for the capitalist, and dividends on shares for shareholders. Goods are always sold for more than the cost of producing them, including the wages of the workers. This will inevitably mean that ordinary workers as a group can never afford all the goods which are available to them—there will be over-production but under-consumption of goods. This is an internal contradiction in capitalism which cannot be resolved, according to Marx.
- ■ Capitalists compete among themselves to make the most profit by selling their goods to the highest number of consumers at the highest price and lowest production cost possible. Consumers are poor (as we just saw) and limited in number. Only production costs are easily altered. To cut these the capitalists will:
  - pay the lowest wages possible (by attacking unions etc);
  - introduce automated production processes.

  The first means that those in work become even poorer. The second means that there will be a large number of people out of work, replaced by machines.
- ■ Those out of work (the 'reserve army of labour') will only be looked after because they may be needed again by the capitalists if new markets are found, or if the old market for their goods picks up again. However within capitalism the Welfare State can and should do no more than this. It is the role of the Welfare State to keep the poor 'ticking over'. To waste any more than the minimum resources on them would:
  - threaten profitability (taxes on profits would increase);
  - make Britain uncompetitive with other capitalist systems abroad. We would be wasting our resources paying to keep the

unemployed and paying higher wages which would put the price of our goods up. Meanwhile they—eg the Koreans—invest their resources in new and better technology while paying minimum wages and not bothering with such niceties as a Welfare State.

From the Marxist perspective, then, it is the structure of capitalism which causes poverty. A system which allows, even encourages, great wealth necessarily creates great poverty. The Marxist would argue that the development of what has been called the 'two nations' in Britain is a consequence of the fact that the government is the ruling committee of the capitalist class. People (predominantly in the North) without work and the hope of getting it, dependent on declining health and welfare services and benefits, are living in a very different world from those (predominantly in the South) in highly paid jobs receiving the benefits of tax cuts and other government measures and who do not use or need the Welfare State. The result has been, and will continue to be, riots in the principle sites of poverty, particularly the inner cities, as those marginalised by the system take matters into their own hands.

☐ **According to the Marxist model:**

- **Who/what is to blame for the existence of poverty?**
- **What needs to be done to abolish it?**
- **Has anything like this been done so far?**

Other conflict perspectives

Many writers on the subject of poverty would agree with Marxists that it results from the conflict over scarce resources between particular groups in society. However such writers would argue that these groups are more specific and numerous than simply two main classes. Peter Townsend is one of these. Adopting a position close to the Weberian one (which sees society as divided up into numerous groups with different levels of status, power and marketable skills and knowledge) Townsend argues that:

> 'There are elaborate rules of professional associations and trade unions, as well as of private firms and public services, including employment agencies and educational institutions, which control access of numbers and social characteristics of individuals ... The form taken by the hierarchy of occupational classes, the differentiated work conditions, status and fringe benefits as well as earnings of those classes, and the institutions controlling access to different levels and sanctioning the conditions associated with each stratum, must comprise a major part of any explanation of poverty.' (*Poverty in the UK*, pp 918–9)

In addition to the different positions within the occupational hierarchy, and differences in the power which groups have to maintain and improve their life chances compared to those of other groups, there are also the people who are outside this hierarchy to consider. These are 'dependants' (children, and housewives, for example) who will either have no income (eg married women) or very low levels of state income. This fact means not only that they are likely to be in poverty, but those people within the occupational hierarchy with a large number of dependants will be too. Other groups are neither employed nor dependants. These people, the retired living alone or in pairs with no private income, the chronically sick, long-term unemployed, single parent families and so on, are particularly likely to be in poverty. They have a very low market situation (ie marketable skills or knowledge) and very little power or status. In the conflict over scarce resources they will be the losers.

Townsend's solution to this situation is listed in six points towards the end of his book:

1. Abolition of excessive wealth (through state policy to restrict it to a maximum permissible level).
2. Abolition of excessive income (by state action to determine top levels of salary).
3. Introducing a more equal income structure and the payment of incomes to dependants to abolish the distinction between earners and dependants.
4. Abolition of unemployment through a legally enforceable right to work.
5. Restrictions on the power and rewards of professions, greater public ownership, more industrial democracy and a stress on cooperation rather than competition at work and in society.
6. More community care for those in need of support so that individuals recognise their responsibilities to others in society.

☐ **What is your response to these suggestions?**

Ingredients of wealth

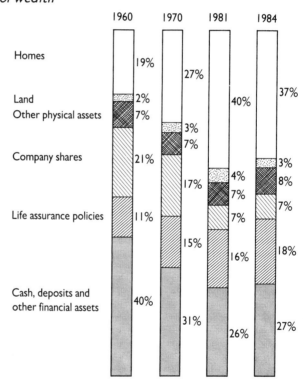

☐ **Use this information to plan how point I of Townsend's proposals could be implemented in practical terms.**

Source: Stark, T. *The A–Z of Wealth*, Table U, The Fabian Society

Functionalists

For the functionalists, Townsend's proposed measures are a recipe for disaster. To writers such as T. Parsons, K. Davis and W. E. Moore and H. Gans it is both inevitable and functional to have very steep gradients in income and wealth with, at the bottom, a reasonably substantial number of poor people.

A steep gradient in the rewards which people are given is inevitable because:

*   everybody is born different, some being more able to do particular things better than others. Some are stronger, others more intelligent, others craftier. Some are good at business, others are good at the arts and so on;

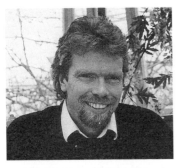

Richard Branson—the self-made man with personal holdings of £149 million in Virgin

☐ **In what ways might Branson be atypical of wealthy people in the UK? What 'socially valued abilities' has he got?**

Generally, what are the arguments against the functionalist view?

☐ **According to the functionalist view, what would be the result of implementing Townsend's proposals 1, 2, 3 and 5?**

☐ **According to the functionalist model:**
  ● **Who/what is to blame for the existence of poverty?**
  ● **What needs to be done to abolish it?**
  ● **Has anything like this been done so far?**

☐ **Divide into groups of about five. You are a policy review committee of a political party (either an established one or a new one). Your tasks are:**

a) **to formulate in writing your general philosophy on poverty in society**
b) **to decide specific policies for the party manifesto.**

● every society considers some abilities good, others less good. This will differ from society to society, but whatever the valued qualities are, they will be rewarded;
● therefore, those lucky enough (say) to be born strong and healthy into a society which values physical strength will find themselves successful and rewarded in it.

It is functional because:

● though people are born with different potential abilities, these need to be developed;
● to encourage people to bother to go through the effort and temporary deprivation of doing this (for example by going to university) there needs to be a high potential reward at the end;
● the higher salaries and fringe benefits attached to the most difficult and most important occupations attract the people with the talent to do them well, and encourage them to develop that talent to the full in order to ensure that they are chosen for the job.

It is inevitable that there is a reasonably substantial number of poor people at the bottom of the social hierarchy because:

● some people will be born without any of the talents that society considers valuable, or perhaps without the self-discipline required to develop them. Such people will not be rewarded.

The existence of poverty is functional because:

● it ensures that the dirty, dead-end jobs in society are done (the poor have no choice);
● it provides jobs for the middle class such as police, probation officers, social workers, psychiatrists and so on;
● it reassures the rest of society by providing an example—'at least I'm not like them', and affirms the value of thrift, hard work, honesty and a stable family life;
● it ensures that shoddy or second-hand goods find a market and that bad or poorly trained professionals can find employment (the poor have to put up with teachers and doctors who can't find employment elsewhere);
● it increases social solidarity among the non-poor by providing a focus for charitable efforts, or (more negatively) providing a folk devil (eg the itinerant poor);
● it both sets the limits of, and legitimates, social norms by providing an example of social situations which are beyond them.

☐ **ESSAY**

1 **'What thoughtful rich people call the problem of poverty, thoughtful poor people call with equal justice the problem of riches.' (R. H. Tawney)**

   a) **Elaborate on what might be meant by this statement. (10 marks)**
   b) **To what extent is it accurate? (15 marks)**

2 **How far have governments since the war succeeded in their aim of eliminating poverty? (25 marks)**

Bibliography

Alcock, P. *Poverty and State Support*, Longman, London 1987

Davis, K. and Moore, W. E. *Some Principles of Stratification* in Bendix, R. and Lipset, S. M. *Class, Status and Power*, RKP 1969

Gans, H. *The Positive Functions of Poverty, American Journal of Sociology 78,* Number 2, 1973

Holman, R. *Poverty: Explanations of Social Deprivation*, Martin Robinson, London 1978

Lewis, O. *The Children of Sanchez*, Penguin, Harmondsworth 1964

Mack, J. and Lansley, S. *Poor Britain*, Unwin Hyman, London 1985

McGregor, S. *The Politics of Poverty*, Longman, London 1981

Rentoul, J. *The Rich Get Richer*, Unwin Hyman, London 1988

Stark, T. *A New A–Z of Income and Wealth*, The Fabian Society, 11 Dartmouth St, London SW1H 9BN

Townsend, P. *Poverty in The United Kingdom*, Penguin, Harmondsworth 1979

Walker, A. and Walker, C. *The Growing Divide*, Child Poverty Action Group, London 1987

The public's perception of necessities

Standard-of-living items in rank order	% classing item as necessity	Standard-of-living items in rank order	% classing item as necessity
1. Heating to warm living areas of the home if it's cold	97	19. A hobby or leisure activity	64
2. Indoor toilet (not shared with another household)	96	20. Two hot meals a day (for adults)	64
3. Damp-free home	96	21. Meat or fish every other day	63
4. Bath (not shared with another household)	94	22. Presents for friends or family once a year	63
5. Beds for everyone in the household	94	23. A holiday away from home for one week a year, not with relatives	63
6. Public transport for one's needs	88	24. Leisure equipment for children, eg sports equipment or a bicycle*	57
7. A warm water-proof coat	87	25. A garden	55
8. Three meals a day for children*	82	26. A television	51
9. Self-contained accommodation	79	27. A 'best outfit' for special occasions	48
10. Two pairs of all-weather shoes	78	28. A telephone	43
11. Enough bedrooms for every child over 10 of different sex to have his/her own*	77	29. An outing for children once a week*	40
12. Refrigerator	77	30. A dressing gown	38
13. Toys for children*	71	31. Children's friends round for tea/a snack once a fortnight*	37
14. Carpets in living rooms and bedrooms	70	32. A night out once a fortnight (adults)	36
15. Celebrations on special occasions such as Christmas	69	33. Friends/family round for a meal once a month	32
16. A roast meat joint or its equivalent once a week	67	34. A car	22
17. A washing machine	67	35. A packet of cigarettes every other day	14
18. New, not second-hand, clothes	64		

Average of all 35 items = 64.1

*For families with children only.

Source: Mack and Lansley, *Poor Britain*, Unwin Hyman 1985 p 54

4 · Health trends and social class in Britain

Occupation unit	Direct age-standardised death rate per 100,000	SMR
University teachers	287	49
Physiotherapists	287	55
Local authority senior officers	342	57
Company secretaries and registrars	362	60
Ministers, senior government officials, MPs	371	61
Office managers	377	64
School teachers	396	66
Architects, town planners	443	74
Civil servants, executive officers	467	78
Medical practitioners	494	81
Coal miners (underground)	822	141
Leather product makers	895	147
Machine tool operators	934	156
Coal miners (above ground)	972	160
Steel erectors, riggers	992	164
Fishermen	1,028	171
Labourers and unskilled workers, all industries	1,247	201
Policemen	1,270	209
Deck and engine room ratings	1,385	233
Bricklayers, labourers	1,644	274

Source: Adapted from Townsend and Davidson (1982) Table 42, p. 194
NB. SMR is Standardised Mortality Ratio. Figures in the second column below 100 indicate a below-average mortality rate and those above 100 an above-average rate.

Health patterns

This chapter is about the patterns of health in Britain. It will first examine trends in health and illness across the country as a whole, and then focus on class structure to examine health inequalities as they are today, and the trends over time.

The good news

The good news about the health of the British population is that generally it is improving over time. This is reflected in many of the figures on health that we have access to:

● The infant mortality rate, thought to be a good indicator of the health of the population as a whole, has fallen from 14.7 in 1975 to 9.1 in 1987.
● Life expectancy has increased. In 1901 a new born baby boy could expect to live for 48 years, a girl for 52. By 1984 this had increased to 72 and 78 respectively.

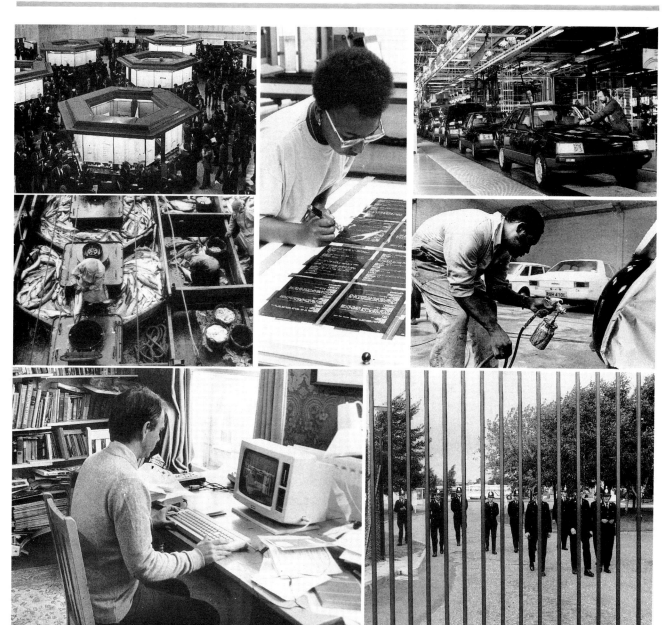

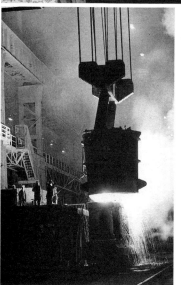

● Certain diseases have been virtually eradicated. These are primarily diseases which are amenable to treatment by immunisation programmes and responsive to improvements in hygiene. They include tuberculosis, typhoid, cholera, diphtheria, meningitis, polio and smallpox. While about one in every 350 people would die each year from tuberculosis in the 1850s, today the figure is one in 100,000. Cholera claimed one in every 550 each year in those days. Today it is wiped out in Britain.
● Pregnancy and childbirth, which in the past were relatively dangerous, now produce few deaths—only 52 in 1984.

It is often thought that it was primarily medical advances such as immunisation that led to the improved health, and decreased death rate, that was a feature of the nineteenth and twentieth centuries in Britain. However, McKeown suggests that the following were far more important (they are in the order of importance which he gives them):

- improved nutrition (resulting from agricultural improvements);
- improvements in hygiene (resulting from better food and water purification, improved sewage disposal, better sterilisation and transport of milk);
- improved environmental conditions (which came later) including improvements in living and working conditions, control of pollution and so on;
- reduced birth rate which restricted numbers so that health improvements could be consolidated.

Document A

'In 1906 Albert Calnette and Camille Guerin discovered a vaccine against the TB germ—it became known as the BCG vaccine ... Vaccines are made from the germs which cause the disease. Once a person has been vaccinated, the body builds up an immunity against these germs and will not catch the disease. Anti-toxins also help fight disease ... When injected into a patient [they] help cure the disease'.

Source: L. Hartley, *History of Medicine*, Basil Blackwell

Document B

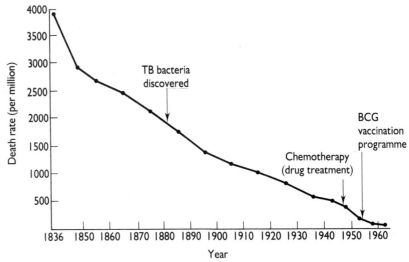

Source: Ibid.

■ **What does the graph tell us about the significance of the BCG vaccination programme?**

The bad news

The bad news is that the incidence of certain types of disease is on the increase in Britain. These include:

- *cancers* of certain types (in just the five years between 1979 and 1984 the numbers of death from cancers of all sorts increased from nearly 130,000 per year to over 140,000). Between 1952 and 1975 there was a 33 per cent increase in mortality from lung cancer. There has been an almost tenfold increase in the number of deaths from cancer in the UK since the middle of the nineteenth century;

- *mental disorder* (between 1979 and 1983 deaths associated with mental disorder increased from 3,211 to 4,142 per year);
- *diabetes* (deaths increased from almost 5,000 in 1979 to nearly 6,500 in 1984);
- *cardiovascular disease* has increased dramatically since the nineteenth century. Today the death rate from heart attacks and strokes in Britain is more than three times higher than it was a hundred years ago;
- *long-standing illness* and illness which limited activity, both in the short and the long term, is being reported by an ever-increasing percentage of the population, (eg 20 per cent of males reporting long-standing illness in 1972 compared to 28 per cent in 1985);
- *degenerative diseases* (those associated with ageing) are on the increase because the number of old people in the population is increasing;
- diseases associated with AIDS (from three cases in the UK in 1982 to over 1,000 deaths in 1988). The Government expects up to 17,000 people to die of AIDS between 1988 and 1992. 10,000 people are known to be infected with HIV, the disease that leads to AIDS after a period of years (five on average), though the real figure is probably nearer 50,000. In the US (where AIDS first became a recognised problem) there were 252 cases in 1981, by December 1985 there were 15,750. Three quarters of all those diagnosed before 1983 had died from their illness by 1985. New York is officially the most AIDS-ridden place in the world. One person in every 1,000 has it (and will die from it). Worldwide, by 1988 a total of 124,000 cases had been reported to the World Health Organisation, though this figure seriously under-represents the real situation. Africa, particularly, has a very serious AIDS problem, but official figures for it are low.

☐ **'*Now there's a cancer to blame on the gays***
It's brutal and fatal and slowly invades,
The Moral Majority like it a lot
'Cause it's the wages of sin and the judgement of God.'
Tom Robinson, *Glad to be Gay* 1987 version © EMI

Put this point into academic language. Use any or all of the following terms: social control, deviance, moral panic, hegemony, folk devils, control culture. (Accounts of S. Cohen's *Folk Devils and Moral Panics*, and S. Hall's *Policing the Crisis* should make these terms clear, as should a dictionary of sociology.)

One fear in the long term is that the tools which medicine uses against disease will stop working. Antibiotics are one of medicine's success stories, yet they are a victim of their own success. Over time, strains of organisms develop which are resistant to antibiotics, and more virulent than previous strains. By providing an environment in which only the strongest organisms can survive, medicine has unwittingly strengthened its 'enemy'. Researchers constantly attempt to develop new types of antibiotics, but these in turn lose their effectiveness, and the number of possible types is not infinite. Doctors are worried that this battle will eventually be lost and that in the future infections will no longer be treatable as they are today. One particularly virulent strain of 'germ' is methicilline-resistant staphylococcus aureus

(MRSA or 'Super Staph'). By 1988 this had been identified in 99 hospitals around Britain and was particularly prevalent in the South East. It is susceptible to only one antibiotic, Vancomycin, which is expensive and toxic. Hospitals are a particularly suitable environment for Super Staph because the widespread use of antibiotics in hospitals kills off other 'germs' and allows Super Staph to proliferate. It is not known how many deaths it has caused, but the elderly and ill are particularly prone to becoming infected with it. One 62 year old female patient died from pneumonia in a London hospital in December 1988 after becoming infected with Super Staph.

More bad news

More disturbing, perhaps, than the failure of medicine to fight some organisms and some sorts of disease, is the fact that some groups in the population, particularly the working class, suffer much worse health than others. Such groups are missing the potential for better health. Let's look at some of the figures about this:

Inequalities in health by social class: the figures

We should not be surprised to find that there are differences in the health and death statistics of the social classes as officially defined. The Registrar General's scheme of social class, based on occupation, was created in order to allow the government to measure differences in the health of different groups in the population. It is as follows:

Social class	Description	Examples	Percentage of economically active and retired males, 1986
I	Professional	Accountant Doctor Lawyer	5
II	Intermediate	Manager School teacher Nurse	18
IIIN	Skilled non-manual	Clerical worker Secretary Shop assistant	12
IIIM	Skilled manual	Bus driver Coal-face worker Carpenter	38
IV	Partly skilled	Agricultural worker Bus conductor Postman	18
V	Unskilled	Labourer Cleaner Dock worker	9

□ **What problems can you see with the Registrar General's scale as a description of the British class structure (there are lots of problems!).**

We will first examine morbidity (ill-health) and then mortality (death) across the class structure.

Morbidity

As we noted earlier, accurate statistics on morbidity are difficult to
come by and are most easily collated from those on mortality.
However, looking at the evidence from a variety of sources including
mortality statistics, the British Heart Survey and the OPCS longitudinal
study we can say that:

- In 65 out of 78 categories of disease in men, the statistics show this
sort of pattern:

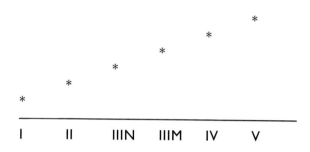

- Only in one category, malignant melanoma (skin cancer caused by
exposure to the sun), is the pattern reversed. However, particular
professions suffer from particular diseases—eg male doctors tend
to suffer more than average from drink-related diseases, as do
journalists.
- In women this pattern applies in 62 out of 82 categories of disease,
with only four showing the reverse (three types of cancer and
malignant melanoma) and the rest evenly spread across the class
structure.
- Individuals in class V and those who are long-term unemployed
have higher blood pressure and tend to be fatter than their class I
counterparts. They are more likely to suffer from arthritis,
haemorrhoids, angina, respiratory problems and deafness. They are
more prone to alcohol-related diseases and mental illness. For
women, mental illness is more likely to be associated with being a
housewife than with being long-term unemployed. If members of
the working class get cancer they are less likely to survive it.
- Children of poor families have more bad teeth and bad lungs than
those in more affluent ones. Respiratory disease and accidents are
the most highly class-related causes of death in children. Children
in social classes IV and V are between five and seven times more
likely to die from accidental death by fire, falling, drowning or
being hit by a motor car than are children from social class I, so we
can assume that accident-related injuries are also closely correlated
with class. Children living in deprived districts of Glasgow were
found to be nine times more likely to be admitted to hospital than
children in non-deprived districts of that city.
- The so-called 'executive diseases' (coronary heart disease, strokes
and peptic ulcers) are now more common in the manual working
class than amongst the executives of class I and II. However, the
'diseases of poverty' (eg cancer of the cervix and tuberculosis)
really are concentrated among the poor and seem likely to remain
so.

- Lower social classes tend to have children of lower birth weight and shorter stature than those of higher social groups. These inequalities seem to continue into adulthood—eg men in the top grades of the civil service are on average five cm taller than those in the lowest grades.
- By the end of the century there would be 100,000 fewer chronically sick and disabled people if health inequalities between social classes were reduced by only 25 per cent.
- Asians living in Britain are more likely to suffer diabetes and coronary heart disease than the white population. Psychiatric illness appears to be more common among Afro-Caribbeans living in Britain than among the population as a whole.

Mortality

- 3,500 children a year would not die if the Infant Mortality Rate of social class V was the same as that of social class I.
- A reduction of 25 per cent in the health inequalities between social classes would produce 20,000 fewer deaths a year in people under pension age in the manual classes.
- Unemployed men and their wives, most of whom come from social class V, have a 20 per cent higher death rate than employed men. Unemployed men are 493 per cent more likely to suffer death related to mental disorders, 503 per cent more of kidney diseases, and 628 per cent more likely to die of 'congenital anomalies' than the national average. Their suicide rate is 173 per cent higher.
- Social class V suffer more from the four biggest killers in Britain than do the higher social groups. These are heart disease, strokes, lung cancer and stomach ulcers.
- The Standardised Mortality Ratio* for males between 15 and 65 is twice as high in social class V as it is in social class I (around 120 compared to around 60).
- The perinatal mortality rate** of babies born in Britain whose mothers are from the West Indies, India, Bangladesh and (particularly) Pakistan, is higher than the national average for all babies, (in 1984, between 14 and 18 per 1,000 babies, depending on the country of origin, compared to an average of 10 per 1,000). Mortality rates from strokes and hypertension are very high among African and Caribbean immigrants, while Asians are more likely than whites to die of coronary heart attacks. Ethnic origin is, of course, related to social class in that most immigrants find themselves in the lower part of the class structure.

To sum up then, we can say that the lower social classes are more likely to suffer from nearly all the major diseases than the higher social classes are, and they are more likely to go to an early grave.

*Standardised Mortality Ratio shows the relative chances of death for a given age. The average SMR for the population of whole of that age is 100, an SMR below this indicates greater 'survivability'.

**Perinatal mortality rate is still births and deaths of infants under one week old per 1,000 live and still births.

The trends

- Between the early 1970s and the early 80s deaths from all causes dropped from an SMR of 100 to 80 for non-manual classes. In manual classes it only declined from 130 to 120.
- In that same decade, deaths from certain diseases have dropped sharply among the non-manual classes but have only dropped slightly or even increased for the manual. These include lung cancer (especially for women) and coronary heart disease.
- The health gap between the social classes is widening as the health of social class I improves at a faster rate than social class V. For example, between 1971 and 1981 there was a 15 per cent overall decline in deaths from heart diseases, but for men and women in non-manual occupations there has been only a 1 per cent decrease.
- The only exception to the generally widening gap in health between the social classes is that class differences in deaths of babies aged between one month and one year narrowed considerably between 1971 and 1981. There has also been a small reduction in differentials between 1 and 4 years (especially for girls).
- The class differential in maternal mortality has remained about the same in recent years.
- Between the end of the 1950s and the beginning of the 1980s there was a decline in the death rate in classes I and II of 37 per cent (for men aged between 45 and 54 years). For men in classes IV and V of that age the decline was only 7 per cent.
- The number of people with long-standing illness in the various classes has increased between 1974 and 1984. This increase is most marked in the lower social classes, so here again the gap is widening.

☐ **Before going on to read the following sections, brainstorm as many reasons as you can which explain the higher mortality and morbidity rates in lower social classes.**

Generally, then, we can say that all classes have profited from a decline in the death rate, but higher status groups have profited the most. However, in the case of certain diseases and long-standing (chronic) illness, there has been an increase in incidence. Here again, the lower social groups have borne the brunt of the increase.

The official response to the statistics on class inequalities

A report on inequalities in health was commissioned by the Labour Government in the late 1970s, and Sir Douglas Black was appointed to head the inquiry. When the Black Report was published in August 1980, the Conservative Government gave it only limited circulation (250 copies) and that after a delay of one year. In a foreword to a Penguin edition of the Report, the then Secretary of State for Social Services stated that he considered implementation of the Report's recommendations would be too expensive and probably ineffective. An update of that Report, entitled *The Health Divide*, was published in March 1987. As had happened to Sir Douglas Black, permission to hold a press conference about the report was refused. The Health Education

Council chair, Sir Brian Bailey, at the last minute prevented the HEC from holding a conference. On 1 April 1987, the HEC was abolished and replaced by the Health Education Authority, with Sir Brian as its chair.

Explanations for inequalities in health

The structural/material explanation

This approach points to factors such as the following to explain the poorer health of the working class:

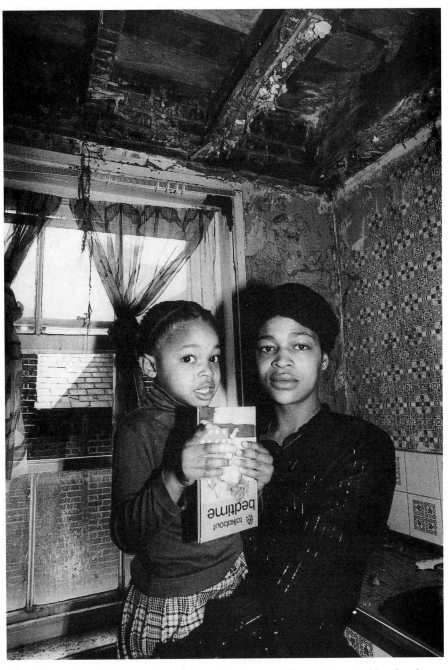

Beveridge's 'giant evil', squalor, is still around in the 1980s, as illustrated by this damp Battersea council flat.

- insufficient household income (leading to poor diet etc)
- unsafe, overcrowded and polluted homes
- cold, damp and unhygienic conditions in the home
- poor communication with the outside world and help agencies
- lack of knowledge and skills in, for example, baby care
- types of working conditions in which accidents are likely
- exposure to hazardous materials at work
- work which is physically and mentally exhausting
- the greater likelihood of severe life events occurring which will then affect health (deaths, poor relationships etc)
- smoking and drinking caused by stress, worry and depression resulting from all the above
- the operation of the 'inverse care law'. This states that: 'the availability of good medical care tends to vary inversely with the need for it in the population served'. (Dr J. Tudor Hart)

☐ **Give specific examples to illustrate how each of the above could lead to disease. How could you test whether they are really a cause of greater ill-health?**

We will examine the last one in some detail. The lack of availability manifests itself in three ways: geographically, in terms of knowledge about facilities, and in the treatment received.

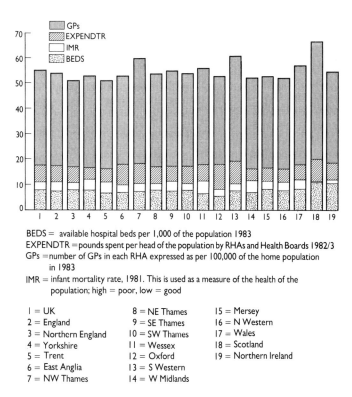

BEDS = available hospital beds per 1,000 of the population 1983
EXPENDTR = pounds spent per head of the population by RHAs and Health Boards 1982/3
GPs = number of GPs in each RHA expressed as per 100,000 of the home population in 1983
IMR = infant mortality rate, 1981. This is used as a measure of the health of the population; high = poor, low = good

1 = UK	8 = NE Thames	15 = Mersey
2 = England	9 = SE Thames	16 = N Western
3 = Northern England	10 = SW Thames	17 = Wales
4 = Yorkshire	11 = Wessex	18 = Scotland
5 = Trent	12 = Oxford	19 = Northern Ireland
6 = East Anglia	13 = S Western	
7 = NW Thames	14 = W Midlands	

Geographical inequalities

Areas where working class people are most numerous tend to be provided with the fewest and worst health facilities. This is despite the fact that working class people suffer worse health than middle class ones and therefore should have more and better facilities. The reasons for this as identified by Hart are as follows:

- Industrial and mining areas have traditionally been serviced by low-status general practitioners, not specialists, hospitals and so on.

- Doctors 'most able to choose where they will work go to middle class areas and ... the areas with highest mortality and morbidity tend to get those doctors who are least able to choose where they will work'. This is partly because 'the better-endowed, better-equipped, better-staffed areas of the service draw to themselves more and better staff, and more and better equipment and their superiority is compounded'.
- 'The career structure and traditions of our medical schools [which] make it clear that time spent at the periphery in the hospital service, or at the bottom of the heap in industrial general practice, is almost certain disqualification for further advancement.'

Inequalities in knowledge

☐ **The quote opposite, and evidence to support these statements, comes from Cartwright and O'Brien. More recently sociologists have come under criticism for making these sorts of statements. It is suggested that, being middle class, sociologists are merely giving vent to their prejudices about the working class. Their studies and results are constructed and interpreted in such a way as to confirm these prejudices. Do you feel that this criticism is valid? How could you objectively test differences between the social classes in these respects?**

People in different social classes behave differently in a medical environment because of the different levels of knowledge they have about it. Those who understand the nature of illnesses, pregnancy and birth control, the facilities available and the procedures for utilising them, will clearly get better service than those who lack such knowledge. Surveys show that middle class people score more highly on questions testing this sort of knowledge than do working class people. Similarly, middle class people are more likely to be critical of any deficiencies in medical service and to demand changes and more information than working class people are. It is suggested that the different social classes *perceive* health facilities in the same way. However the working class are more diffident about expressing their views:

'Patients in the professional class were more likely to ask questions, while those in the unskilled manual group more often waited to be told'.

Middle class people are especially able to use this knowledge to take advantage of the facilities for preventive services. They therefore have a pro-active rather than a re-active approach to health, (ie preventing health problems from arising rather than simply responding to them once they appear).

Differential treatment by professionals

Doctors and other professionals behave differently when dealing with people from different social groups. Studies show that middle class patients are given *longer* consultations by doctors (about six minutes compared to just over four for the working class). More problems are discussed during the middle class consultation (about four compared to about three)—though the ratio of 'social' as opposed to 'medical' problems is about the same for the two groups.

Middle class people are more likely to ask questions, as we saw above, and though they may get cut short by the doctor, this is more likely to happen if the patient is working class. Doctors are more likely to know the names and domestic situations of their middle class patients than their working class ones, despite the fact that the working class patients are more likely to have been with the practice longer. This not only applies to social class. Black patients have been found to talk more to a psychiatrist if they share the same ethnic background. White psychiatrists appear more likely to classify black patients as mentally disturbed than white patients. This is because, as Hart suggests, doctors are most frequently drawn from the ranks of the white middle class (and are often the children of doctors) so they find if difficult to empathise with other social groups.

General practice consultations with middle and working class patients aged 65 and over

	Middle class	Working class
Average length of consultation (min)	6.2	4.7
Average number of questions asked by patient	3.7	3.0
Average number of problems discussed	4.1	2.8
Average number of symptoms mentioned to interviewer prior to consultation	2.2	3.0

Source: adapted from Cartwright, A. and O'Brien, M., *Social Class Variations in Health Care and in General Practitioner Consultations*, in *The Sociology of the NHS*, Sociological Review Monograph no. 22, Stacey, M., (ed.), University of Keele, 1976.

□ **Assuming we would want equality of opportunity for all social groups in the medical situation, what policies could we implement to bring this about? (Deal with each of the three categories above—inequalities in resources, knowledge and treatment by professionals.)**

The artefact explanation—more good news?

An 'artefact' is something that is made by people, is artificial rather than natural. This explanation says that the 'bad news' about class and health is not really true—it only appears to be the case because of artificial and inaccurate statistics. The statistics are wrong because:

- The percentage of people in the lower social groups is declining all the time. Eventually there could be a situation in which there were only one or two people in social class V, yet it would still be possible to talk about 'the health divide'. In fact, as this class disappears, so does the reality of the health divide.

□ **Why are social classes IV and V disappearing?**

- Even for those who remain in the lower social groups, the general level of health is improving. In some types of illness the rate of improvement is greater in the lower social groups than the higher. These facts shouldn't be forgotten.
- Arguments about the health divide are usually based on figures which relate only to males of working age. If females and older and younger people were taken into account then many aspects of the divide would be shown to be artificial. For example the higher social groups are more likely to suffer from the degenerative diseases which affect older people more (higher social classes live longer and so have more older people among their number).

□ **In reply to the last point, the authors of *Inequalities in Health* argue that using social class defined in this way probably *under*estimates the degree of health inequalities, if anything. How would you reply to the other points?**

- Organising the statistics in terms of 'social class', defined in terms of the job of the breadwinner in the family, is meaningless. There are many much more meaningful ways of classifying people and their diseases (for example by income, by ownership of assets, by social isolation, by overcrowding and so on). Therefore the results of such arbitrary classification are meaningless too.

The social selection explanation

This explanation argues that people in poor health tend to move to or stay in the bottom of the occupational scale or the ranks of the unemployed *because* of their poor health. It isn't that they have poor

☐ **What sort of evidence would you need to collect in order to confirm or refute this idea?**

health because they're in classes IV and V, rather they are in classes IV and V because of their poor health. The fact that people at higher levels of the civil service are taller than their lower status colleagues is easily explained. Psychologists have shown that taller people get better jobs because people perceive them more positively than shorter ones. But you don't need to be a psychologist to realise that someone who is frequently ill and takes time off school or work is less likely to succeed than someone who is healthy and in full possession of their faculties during their period of education and at work.

The behavioural/cultural explanation

The explanation blames those with ill-health for not looking after themselves properly. The cause lies in unhealthy behaviour such as smoking and drinking too much, not taking enough exercise, eating the wrong sorts of foods and so on. Not only is their behaviour inclined to make them less healthy, they are less likely to bother to make use of facilities provided to keep them healthy, for instance by going for medical check-ups, using family planning facilities and so on. These habits are often transmitted across the generations in the process of socialisation and could therefore be said to be part of the 'culture of poverty' (see page 49).

In the autumn of 1986 the Under-Secretary of State for Health, Edwina Currie, said that the real cause of the poorer health of Northerners is their diet. Ill-health could best be tackled by:

'Impressing upon people the need to look after themselves better'.

Despite much criticism of her outspoken comments on this theme, she continued to expound it:

'Don't eat the pud! There's no law that says you've got to eat everything that's under your nose'.

(These quotes are part of the advice given to businessmen and women in *Your Business*, July 1988 p 19.)

Lower social classes and the unemployed tend to smoke and drink more and to take less exercise—all causes of high cholesterol levels and heart problems which they suffer from more than other groups. Low income families eat more unhealthy food like processed meat and fried meals. They buy fewer fresh vegetables and healthy fibre-rich foods.

It's never too late to start looking after your heart. You can reduce your risk of heart disease by making just a few simple changes.

Heart disease is the most common cause of death in Britain today. It kills more people than all the different types of cancer put together. Although men are even more at risk than women, it is also a major problem for women.

There is no single cause of heart disease. In most cases it is caused by several factors, all working together. But take heart. There is a lot you can do to avoid some of these factors and reduce your risk of heart disease.

'A few simple changes' in your behaviour can reduce your risk of heart disease, according to the behavioural-cultural point of view.

Table 1: The relationship between smoking and employment, 1984

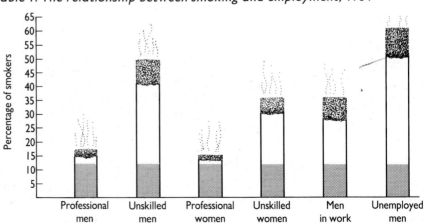

☐ **To test the cultural/behavioural explanation, develop a questionnaire concerning people's eating, drinking and smoking habits. Also, ask them about their attitudes to and knowledge of food and health (eg by setting them test questions about which are 'healthy' and 'unhealthy' foods.) By asking them about their age, occupation and so on, you can determine whether there is any correlation between these and the factors tested.**

They have larger families too, which means greater danger of infection, and fewer resources for each child.

Respiratory diseases in children have been shown to be highly related to parents' smoking, and the risk of infection increases with the size of the family. Thus the class-related nature of this illness can be explained by the patterns of behaviour of parents in lower social groups. Similarly the larger number of fatal accidents to children in the lower social groups is explained by their greater carelessness, lower levels of parental supervision and general macho attitudes towards danger.

The structural approach, which says that the lower social groups are forced into certain forms of behaviour by their low income and poor environments, is nonsense. You need to have money to smoke and drink. If social class V followed the example of class I and moderated this behaviour they could afford to feed their children better (especially if they had fewer of them). Going for a regular two mile walk in order to become fitter costs nothing, yet only 13 per cent of class V did it in 1983 compared to 30 per cent of class I. Indoor swimming costs very little, yet the figures were 3 and 12 per cent respectively.

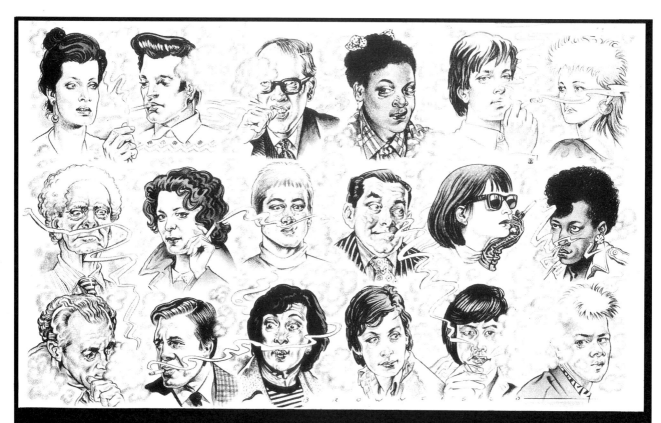

Only one out of every three people smokes.
The other two choke.

Don't force your smoke down other people's throats.

The way to create a healthier Britain? The HEAs attempt to change people's behaviour.

Stress as an explanation of inequalities in health

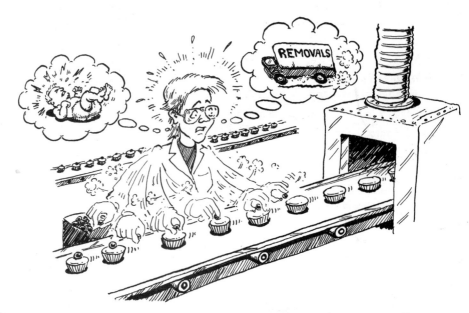

Heading for an early grave? Highly stressed, and possibly a smoker too.

This explanation argues that the lower social groups are more likely to suffer stress and this makes them more prone to disease. For example, people living in noisy and dangerous environments who have stressful or insecure jobs will be at risk. So will those whose jobs are boring and repetitive. The BMA thinks stress may be a significant factor in why black immigrants to Britain suffer worse health than the host population.

Studies into the effects of stress demonstrate that important events in a person's life can provoke illnesses of various kinds, both physical and mental. For example, bereavement, redundancy, retirement or the failure of one's plans have been shown to be frequently followed by depressive illness or gastro-intestinal disease. The mechanisms causing this are associated with the immune system (so that the person cannot throw off disease), and elements of the nervous and chemical systems of the body.

Genetic differences as an explanation of inequalities in health

This explanation argues that the lower social groups are *genetically* more prone to certain types of disease, and less resistant to others, than the higher social groups. Research by Dr Beardmore has shown that lower social groups are more likely to have blood group O, though what the significance of this may be is not known. Asians in Britain have higher levels of cardiovascular disease than is found in other groups. This is despite the fact that typical Asian food is 'healthier' in this respect than typical 'British' food. The BMA suggests that genetic differences between Asians and the native British might be the cause of the higher levels of heart disease among the Asians. Another genetic difference, in skin pigmentation, results in white Australians being very prone to skin cancer, while Aborigines are very unlikely to suffer from it.

□ **What methodology/ies could you employ to test the relationship between stress and ill-health?**

□ **How might genetic differences between social classes in Britain arise? Do you consider this a likely explanation? Why/why not?**

□ **Take one of the six explanations for the health divide and consider what social policies could be employed in each case in order to narrow it.**

□ **ESSAY**

'While the rich and the poor are both getting healthier, the gap between them in health terms is getting wider.'

What evidence is there in support of this statement and how can the widening gap be explained?

Bibliography

Black, N. *Health and Disease: A Reader*, Open University Press, Milton Keynes 1984

BMA, *Deprivation and Ill-Health*, 1987, available from the BMA, Tavistock Square, London WC1H 9JP (has a good bibliography)

Cartwright, A. and O'Brien, M. *Social Class Variations in Health Care and in the Nature of General Practice Consultations*, in Tuckett, D. and Kaufert, J. M. *ibid*, pp 89–97

Doll, R. and Peto, R. *The Causes of Cancer*, Oxford University Press, Oxford 1981

Gibson, I. *Class, Health and Profit*, University of East Anglia, Norwich 1981

Green, J. and Miller, D. *Aids: The Story of a Disease*, Grafton Books, London 1986

Hart, J. T. *The Inverse Care Law*, Lancet, Volume 1: pp 405–12, 1971

Hart, N. *The Sociology of Health and Medicine*, Causeway Press, Ormskirk 1985

Heller, T. *Poor Health, Rich Profits*, Spokesman Books, London 1977

McKeown, T. *The Role of Medicine*, Basil Blackwell, Oxford 1979

Mitchell, J. *What Is To Be Done About Illness and Health?*, Penguin, Harmondsworth 1984

New Scientist, Its the Poor What Get the Disease, 7 August 1986

Office of Population Censuses and Surveys, *The General Household Survey*, 1985, HMSO London 1987

Patrick, D. L. and Scambler, G. (eds), *Sociology as Applied to Medicine*, Balliere Tindall, Eastbourne 1986 (2nd edition)

Richman, J. *Medicine and Health*, Longman, London 1987

Silverman, D. *Medical Sociology*, Sage, London 1988

Townsend, P., Davidson, N. and Whitehead, M. *Inequalities in Health*, Penguin, Harmondsworth 1988 (2nd edition)

Trowler, P. *Topics in Sociology*, Unwin Hyman, London 1984 (for accounts of studies on stress, pp 206–7)

Tuckett, D. and Kaufert, J. M. *Basic Readings in Medical Sociology*, Tavistock Publications, London 1978

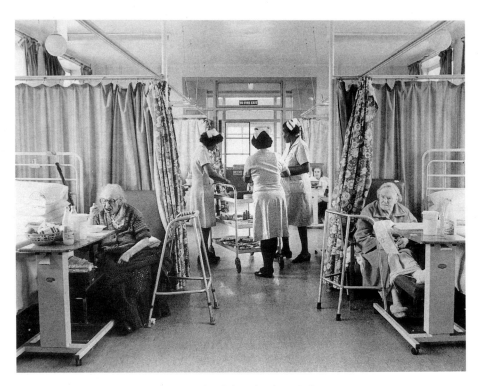

Making welfare work—women in a North London hospital.

This chapter will first examine the evidence about and explanations of gender inequalities in health, both within the UK and abroad. It will then go on to examine the role of women in health and welfare work.

Morbidity, mental illness and gender

- In 1985 14 per cent of women compared to 11 per cent of men reported acute health problems (ie illness or injury which restricted their activity in the two weeks prior to being interviewed). The gender differential had increased compared to 1972, when it was only 8 per cent and 7 per cent respectively.
- 29 per cent of men but 31 per cent of women reported having chronic sickness (ie a long-standing illness, disability or infirmity).
- Of these, 16 per cent of men but 18 per cent of women reported their chronic sickness to be so severe as to limit their activity.
- Women see their doctor more frequently than men: five times a year compared to three times a year in 1985.
- In 1985, 11 per cent of females compared to 8 per cent of males had been a patient in hospital in the previous 12 months.
- Two thirds of the four million disabled people in the UK are women.
- 57 per cent of admissions to mental hospitals (for any disorder) are women. However, women are even more likely than men to be admitted for certain types of mental illness, particularly:
  - emotional disturbance;

- neurotic disorders;
- depression;
- senile dementia.
- Men equal women in the number of admissions for schizophrenia and paranoia, and have a much greater admission rate for alcohol dependence.
- One in five women suffers acute stress or depression according to the Government's advisory *Women's National Commission*. In a report (published in July 1988) they say that women are twice as likely to suffer severe stress as men because they tend to be 'the buffer and absorber of stresses of the other members of the family'. Women cope by turning stress in on themselves, and this often leads to alcohol or cigarette addiction. Women are more likely than men to become heavy and dependent drinkers following stressful events such as marital breakdown.

Mortality and gender

Table 1 Selected causes of death by sex and age, 1951 and 1984

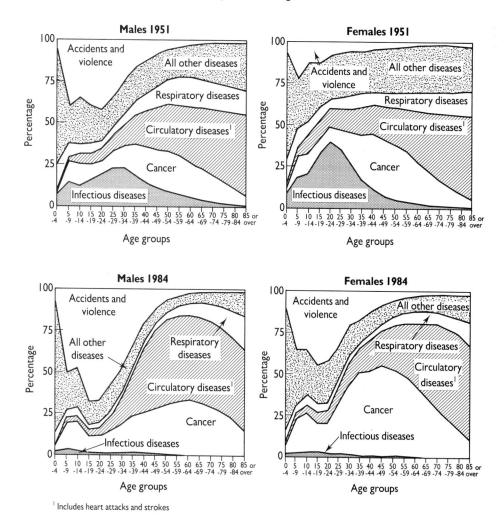

1 Includes heart attacks and strokes

Source: Social Trends, 1987

☐ **From Table I on p. 73, identify:**

- **changes in the causes of death between 1951 and 1981;**
- **differences in the causes of death between men and women.**

What possible explanations might there be for the trends and differences you have identified?

- Life expectancy at birth in the UK is 77 years for females but 71 for males (1988).
- As a result around 70 per cent of those over 75 are women, this percentage increasing for older age-groups.
- The number of stillborn male babies is consistently greater than females (1,983 compared to 1,662 in 1985). Though there are more male babies born than females, this does not account for the greater number of stillbirths. The percentage of stillbirths compared to live births in 1985 was 0.588 per cent for males but 0.5200 per cent for females. The rates of miscarriages and neonatal deaths, as well as the infant mortality rate, are also higher for boys than girls.
- The gap between women and men has been increasing in Britain— the improvements in life expectancy have benefited women more than men (largely because of a great decline in deaths during childbirth).

Table 2 Top 20 causes of death in 1976, death rates per million population, in England and Wales.

Females	Rate	Males	Rate
1. Cerebrovascular disease	1,851	1. Acute myocardial infarction	2,678
2. Acute myocardial infarction	1,686	2. Cerebrovascular disease	1,200
3. Pneumonia	1,263	3. Cancer of trachea, bronchus and lung	1,110
4. Myocardial degeneration	992	4. Myocardial degeneration	1,051
5. Cancer of breast	466	5. Pneumonia	994
6. Cancer of trachea, bronchus and lung	275	6. Bronchitis	717
7. Arteriosclerosis	262	7. Cancer of stomach	289
8. Cancer of large intestine except rectum	251	8. Cancer of prostate	192
9. Bronchitis	239	9. Cancer of large intestine except rectum	186
10. Cancer of stomach	196	10. Motor vehicle traffic accidents	171
11. Hypertensive disease	168	11. Aortic aneurysm (non-syphilitic)	152
12. Influenza	165	12. Hypertensive disease	142
13. Chronic rheumatic heart disease	148	13. Cancer of rectum	139
14. Cancer of ovary, fallopian tube and broad ligament	147	14. Arteriosclerosis	138
15. Cancer of uterus	146	15. Cancer of bladder	123
16. Accidental falls	130	16. Cancer of pancreas	119
17. Diabetes mellitus	120	17. Influenza	106
18. Cancer of rectum	116	18. Suicide	97
19. Cancer of pancreas	110	19. Chronic rheumatic heart disease	87
20. Aortic aneurysm (non-syphilitic)	83	20. Diabetes mellitus	86
All causes	11,829	All causes	12,527

From OPCS (1983).

Source: D. L. Patrick and G. Scambler, *Sociology as applied to Medicine.*

The attentive student may notice an apparent paradox here: women suffer from worse health than men, yet they live longer! The possible explanations for how they manage to pull off this particular trick are:

- though women suffer more ill-health, the predominantly male forms of ill-health are more fatal (eg emphysema, heart disease, arteriosclerosis);
- men enjoy generally better health than women but are killed off by accidents and diseases which they are more susceptible to and which are often fatal;
- women suffer worse health precisely *because* they live longer—ie from the degenerative diseases associated with old age;
- the statistics on morbidity or mortality or both are wrong in some way.

There seems to be some truth in each of these, as we shall see below.

Statistics abroad

Mortality

☐ **What hypotheses can you formulate to explain the higher death rate of females in these four countries only? Think of at least three.**

How could your hypotheses be tested:

a) given unlimited resources;
b) given the resources you actually have?

☐ **Develop some hypotheses to explain these figures.**

- Life expectancy at birth, while generally lower in low-income economies (around 50 years), still favours females. In 1984, women could expect to live longer than men in all but four of the 36 underdeveloped countries identified by the World Bank. Interestingly, these four are close neighbours—India, Pakistan, Nepal and Bhutan.
- In none of the other 92 countries above this level of development was there a higher life expectancy for men than for women. Only Iran had an equal life expectancy at birth for males and females (61 years).
- The average advantage in life expectancy which females had over males (calculating from the time they were born) in 1984 was:
  - one year in low income economies
  - four years in middle income economies
  - five years in upper-middle income economies
  - six years in industrial market economies.
- Comparing the gap between male and female life expectancies at birth in 1965 with that in 1984:
  - the average for low income countries has reduced by one year
  - in middle income ones it has increased by one year
  - in upper-middle income ones it has increased by one year
  - in industrial-market economies it has remained constant at six years.
- In East European socialist economies, the gap between male and female life expectancy at birth was five years (66 years as against 71 years) in 1984. In none of the eight countries in this category was male expenctancy greater than 69 years or female less than 74 years. The male/female life expectancy gap had reduced by two years between 1965 and 1984 in these countries.

Why are there sex differences in morbidity and mortality?

☐ **In Chapter 4 we looked at the following explanations for the inequalities in health of the different social classes:**

- **social-structural/material**
- **artefact**
- **social selection**
- **behavioural/cultural**
- **stress**
- **genetic differences**

Try applying the same types of explanation (excluding the third, which does not apply here) to the inequalities in health of the sexes—the greater morbidity of some types among women and the higher mortality rates among men. (Do this *before* reading the following sections!)

The social-structural/material explanation

Women's position in society shapes their experience of health and health care. The health-threatening aspects of women's role in Western industrialised society include the following:

- the burden of child care
- the demands of looking after other people's health
- the demands of domestic labour
- poor employment conditions (low pay, insecure and part-time work)
- greater exposure to poor housing
- greater exposure to poverty

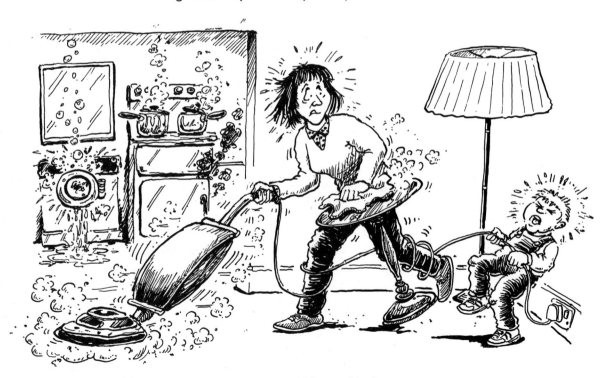

Not at work . . . or just not paid for working?

Jessie Bernard is well known for her studies of the unhealthy nature of housework. In *The Wife's Marriage*, she identifies 'the housewife syndrome', the symptoms of which are nervousness, inertia, insomnia, nightmares and so on. The housewife is more prone to these symptoms than, for example, the working woman. Generally she finds that while the single woman is healthier than the married woman, the single man is less healthy than the married one. Thus getting married and giving up paid work can damage your health (if you are a woman). Perhaps there should be a government health warning on the marriage certificate.

The genetic explanation for higher levels of morbidity (see below) is undermined by the following facts:

- There have been times in British history when female death rates were higher than males (in 1846 among 25–34 year olds, and in 1896 among 5–14 year olds). Similarly, in four countries women live less long than men (though presumably their biology is virtually identical to that of women elsewhere).
- Heart disease among younger females is now on the increase, which raises questions about the validity of the oestrogen-protection argument (see p 80).

□ **In what ways could the gender differentials in health be reduced?**

The artefact explanation

This argues that women don't really suffer worse health than men, but the statistics make it appear that they do for the following reasons:

- Often the statistics only relate to one variable (in the case of the figures above it is sex). This can be misleading. For example, women who are in low social classes and/or ethnic minorities are doubly disadvantaged in terms of health, as well as in other ways. For instance, in 1985 41 per cent of women in social class V were suffering from a long-standing illness. The average for all women, though, was 31 per cent. If age too is taken into account, we find, for example, that social class V men between the ages of 45 and 64 suffer more chronic illness than females of the same age group and social class. Thus, the variables we choose, and those we omit, can alter what the statistics appear to show. As women are disproportionately represented in particular occupational categories and age groups, these may be the important factors, not sex.
- Often the figures do not tell us what we want to know. For example, do women visit the doctor more frequently than men because they suffer more ill-health, or for some other reason?
- Statistics based on surveys can be inaccurate because of high non-response rates, and the practice of proxy reporting for men (ie wives fill in the form, even the sections relating to the man's health and medical history).
- Statistics on morbidity are notoriously inaccurate because of the clinical iceberg. We cannot be sure about the facts of gender-related differences in morbidity because women may, for example, be more willing to adopt the sick role than men (or, conversely, be more inclined to 'soldier on'). Similarly self-report studies (eg the question 'have you suffered incapacitating illness in the last 24 days?' asked by the General Household Survey) are also unreliable.

□ **What other reasons might there be for women visiting the doctor more frequently than men?**

The cultural/behavioural explanation

This argues that men do things which are so seriously health-threatening that they are likely to die from them. For example they eat the wrong foods, and smoke and drink more than women. Generally, they are less aware of the health of their body and the importance of balanced eating etc.

- Well over half the difference between the male and female death rate can be accounted for by differences in behaviour (eg cigarette smoking, alcohol consumption and occupational hazards, suicide and traffic accidents).

Table 3 Some selected forms of unhealthy behaviour

	Males	Females
% describing themselves as 'heavier drinker' (GB 1984)	20%	2%
% smokers (GB 1984)	36%	32%
Average number of cigarettes smoked per week	115	96
Admissions to hospital for drug dependence (GB 1985)	2,862	1,522

Some health consequences of dangerous or unhealthy behaviour

	Males	Females
Malignant cancers of the lung, bronchea, pleura and trachea (associated with smoking) (England and Wales 1982)	27,446	9,441
Diseases of the respiratory system (patients in hospital) (England and Wales 1984)	237,200	186,400
% of deaths caused by accidents and violence at 18 years old (GB 1984)	70%	45%

Sources: Social Trends, 1988, and *Health and Personal Social Services Statistics for England and Wales*, 1986.

This perspective can also explain the worse morbidity of women:

- Women are socialised into an unhealthy set of norms and values. They willingly take on responsibilities which make them prone to physical and mental disorder. These include those listed on pages 72–74, but here the emphasis is on women's *choice* in doing these things. The social-structural explanation suggests that they are victims of social and economic circumstance.

The stress explanation

Modern medicine now realises that the level of stress one is subject to can affect one's resistance to disease. Stress may take the form of constant pressure on the individual resulting from their environment, work, family or social circumstances. Alternatively it may come in short but powerful bursts related to specific life events such as bereavement, divorce, and so on. In either case the health effects can be devastating. It is thought that, compared to men, women are particularly subject to stress for the reasons outlined below.

- The 'housewife syndrome' (see above) appears to be associated with stress. Bernard and other feminists argue that the isolation and constant decision-making involved in housework is very stressful to the women who do it, as is the responsibility of caring for a young child.

- Women act as the absorber of stresses of other family members. Functionalists argue that women play the 'affective' (emotional) role in the family and make it into a haven for the 'instrumental' male to recover from the demands of the wider world. Functionalists do not appreciate, though, that adopting the role of counsellor and therapist for the rest of the family make demands upon the women themselves.

The social situation in which women are placed in most societies means that they take the burden of stress. In this context, then, stress is related to social structure. This explanation is therefore part of the social structural/material explanation.

☐ **Read Cline and Spender's *Reflecting Men at Twice Their Natural Size*. Do you agree with their account of the role women play in inflating men's egos for them?**

The genetic explanation

Women suffer from certain sorts of health problems because of their distinctive biology—ie things which it is impossible for men to suffer from. This includes things associated with:

- pregnancy and childbirth
- contraception and abortion
- menstruation and menopause
- breast and cervical cancer

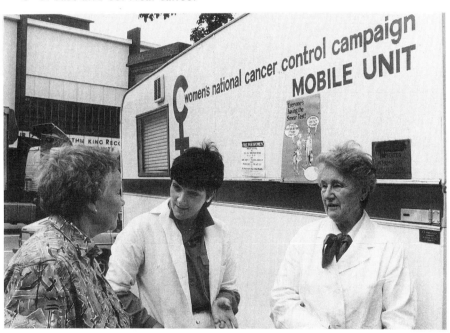

Caring for women in London; cancer control organised by Lambeth's Health Authority and Borough Council

In addition there are certain illnesses which women are more likely to suffer from than men because of their different biology:

- Because women have a greater immune response than men they suffer far more from auto-immune diseases which occur when the body's defence system attacks a substance which is part of one's body, rather than a foreign substance. Arthritis is one of these, and affects women three times more frequently than men.

- Because women live longer than men they are more likely to suffer from the 'degenerative diseases'—ie those associated with ageing.

Men, too, suffer from some types of worse health and have a higher mortality rate generally, because of genetic factors:

- Men suffer more heart disease because they lack the oestrogen hormones which offer protection against it and which are present in women until the menopause at around 50, when women begin to suffer an equal risk of heart disease.
- There is some evidence that the chromosome difference in men and women has an effect. Men normally have one X and one Y chromosome, while women have two Xs. A study of four generations of an Amish family in Pennsylvania showed that males who were missing the long arm of their Y chromosomes substantially outlived the women. However, in two neighbouring Amish families where the men had normal Y chromosomes (ie no deletion), the mortality pattern was normal—women outlived men.
- Death rates are greater among males even before social factors have had a chance to come into play—eg the rate of stillbirths, perinatal mortality etc. This shows that genetic rather than social factors are important.

□ **What criticisms do you have of the methodology of this study?**

Women and welfare

L. Balbo in an article called '*Crazy Quilts*' uses the metaphor of patchwork quilts to discuss women's role in health and welfare. She says that women, through their servicing work in the home and in the NHS, social services and so on, hold modern society (the quilt) together. Society comprises a disorganised and complex array of fragmentary institutions, with inadequate resources. Yet it hangs together thanks to the labour of women, largely unpaid, usually unrecognised and always undervalued.

> 'They [women] patch together resources to meet human needs ... This packaging of resources requires intelligence, planning, creativity, time and hard work. And just as in a patchwork quilt, the end result is design, logic and order.' (p 24)

One example of this happening is in the policy of 'community care' (see pages 102–103). Though apparently well organised, in practice it means that the burden of care for the sick and the elderly falls predominantly on women. This is neatly summed up in the formula:

community care = family care = care by women

□ **Consider the effects on the woman, and on the relationships within the family, of caring for a disabled elderly relative in her home. If possible prepare a structured interview schedule about this issue and conduct one or more interviews with female carers whom you know.**

It is estimated that there are 1.3 million people acting as the principle carers to disabled adults and children. Probably three-quarters of these are women; the wives, mothers, sisters, daughters and daughters-in-law of the disabled person. At any one time 20 per cent of women between 40 and 59 will be providing such care, and probably half of all women will do so at some stage in their lives. 6.5 million parents act as the primary carer of children under the age of 16 years, and in 95 per cent of households it is the mother who is the principal carer.

Professionally, too, women tend to work in the caring professions,

☐ **Official estimates suggest that informal care by females in the home will be less likely to occur in the future, despite the increasing number of old people in the population, and the Government's desire for more community care. Why might this be so?**

especially in the lower parts of those professions. The NHS is the single biggest employer of women in this country—three quarters of its employees are female. Yet these are not spread evenly through the hierarchical structure of the NHS:

- 75 per cent of ancillary workers (cleaners, cooks etc) are female
- 86 per cent of nurses are female
- 20 per cent of full-time GPs are female

Hospital medical staff, England, 1985

Grade	Females as a percentage of total in grade
Consultant and Senior House Medical Officer	23
Associate specialist	12.5
Senior Registrar	23
Registrar	21
Senior House Officer	32
House Officer	39

Source: adapted from *Health and Personal Social Services Statistics For England, 1986*, HMSO 1986

Even within these categories there are male and female specialisms. Consultants in child and adolescent psychiatry and mental handicap are about ten times more likely to be women than those in any type of surgery. Elsewhere within the NHS, too, there are gender-based specialisms:

- male nurses are concentrated in psychiatric nursing;
- female doctors and consultants tend to specialise in obstetrics, paediatrics etc;
- only five out of the 16,000 midwives in England are male.

Outside the NHS we find that:

- 80 per cent of the staff in old-people's homes are women;
- 75 per cent of the staff in children's homes are women;
- most primary school teachers are women, but few Heads are;
- most social workers on lower grades are women;
- women figure prominently in voluntary organisations such as Help the Aged, the Red Cross and so on. Their work is either free or low paid.

Women and medicine

Feminists are critical of the biomedical approach over a number of issues, though fundamentally they all revolve around the point that biomedicine is controlled by men who use their power to the detriment of women's interests. This patriarchal medical practice is most evident in the following areas:

- pregnancy and childbirth;
- contraception.

Pregnancy and childbirth

Hilary Graham and Ann Oakley show how the view held about the nature of childbirth by obstetricians on the one hand, and mothers on the other, are quite different and lead to conflict. For the obstetrician, childbirth is a medical problem, indistinguishable from other aspects of medical work. Women and their babies are 'cases' and need to be 'dealt with' efficiently (and according to the needs of the hospital—inducing the baby's birth at a convenient time if necessary). Women, on the other hand, see childbirth as natural, not medical, and as an experience to be savoured rather than got through quickly. Women desire control over the process and over their own bodies, but this is denied by doctors who are in the position to exert control.

Contraception

Feminists note how the technology of contraception has been directed at the female far more than the male. The only commonly available form of contraception for the male, the sheath, has no possibility of harmful side effects. Yet every other form, all of which are used by the female, can have harmful effects on the health of women. The negative effects of Western (and male dominated) medicine are confined to women where possible. Contraceptive pills can cause cancer, IUDs and the cap can make women susceptible to infections and other complications. Depo provera (an injectable contraceptive) has been banned in the United States because of its side effects, but is still used elsewhere in the world, including Britain. Even ancient civilisations gave women a fairly hard time in this area. The ancient Egyptians used crocodile dung pessaries, while the Middle East used camel dung ones. The Ancient Greeks and Romans simply killed their unwanted new-born girls. Hebrew women in the time of Christ used sponges dipped in brandy or vinegar.

Women and social policy

Feminists argue that 'welfare' legislation has incorporated the patriarchal ideology of the society that originated it. Acts such as the Factory Acts of the nineteenth century, which were supposedly designed to protect women from working long hours in unsafe conditions, in fact were designed to take them out of the workforce and keep them in the home, no longer competing with men for jobs. The 1911 National Insurance Act insured male workers but excluded married women, who were thought to be the responsibility of their husband and dependent on him. The Beveridge Report adopted the same approach: 'the attitude of the housewife to gainful employment outside the home is not and should not be the same as that of the single woman. She has other duties ...'. Women in part-time jobs today are often excluded from welfare benefits because they are not covered by the National Insurance system. Similarly they may find themselves denied non-contributory benefit because, as a result of their child-care responsibilities, they find they are defined as 'not available for work' by the local benefit office. This makes them ineligible for benefit. Until a ruling by the European Court in the mid 1980s, it was the case that while men (married or single) and single women could claim benefit for caring for an invalid relative in the home, married women could not. The thinking was that this was part of their normal duties and should not be subsidised by the state. Even today, then, there is still a reluctance to integrate women fully into the welfare state, and, indeed, a reluctance to go too far in replacing the unpaid work of women within the family by welfare institutions. Patrick Jenkin illustrated this neatly when he was Secretary of State for the Social Services:

'There is now elaborate machinery to ensure that [women have] equal opportunity, equal pay and equal rights but I think we ought to stop and ask "where does this leave the family"?'.

☐ **Read the account below of a new penile device designed as a contraceptive for men.**

What points are being made by this spoof article?

The newest development in male contraception was unveiled recently at the American Women's Surgical Symposium held at the Ann Arbor Medical Center. Dr Sophie Merkin of the Merkin Clinic announced the preliminary findings of a study conducted on 763 unsuspecting male undergraduates at a large Midwestern university. In her report, Dr Merkin stated that the new contraceptive—the IPD—was a breakthrough in male contraception. It will be marketed under the trade name 'Umbrelly'.

The IPD (intrapenile device) resembles a tiny rolled umbrella which is inserted through the head of the penis and pushed into the scrotum with a plunger-like device. Occasionally there is perforation of the scrotum, but this is disregarded as the male has few nerve endings in this area of his body. The underside of the umbrella contains a spermicidal jelly, hence the name 'Umbrelly'.

Experiments on 1,000 white whales from the continental shelf (whose sexual apparatus is said to be closest to man's) proved the IPD to be 100 per cent effective in preventing the production of sperm, and eminently satisfactory to the female whale since it does not interfere with her rutting pleasure.

Dr Merkin declared the umbrelly to be statistically safe for the human male. She reported that of the 763 undergraduates tested with the device only two died of scrotal infection, only 20 developed swelling of the testicles, and 13 were too depressed to have an erection. She stated that common complaints ranged from cramping and bleeding to acute abdominal pains. She emphasised that these symptoms were merely indications that the man's body had not yet adjusted to the device. Hopefully the symptoms would disappear within a year.

☐ **ESSAY**

'Both present patterns and historical trends in health and illness can only be understood in the context of social and economic systems'. Discuss this statement with particular reference to the different patterns of health and illness among men and women.

One complication caused by the IPD and briefly mentioned by Dr Merkin was the incidence of massive scrotal infection necessitating the surgical removal of the testicles. 'But this is a rare case', said Dr Merkin, 'too rare to be statistically important'. She and other distinguished members of the Women's College of Surgeons agreed that the benefits far outweighed the risk to any individual man. [From *Outcome* magazine, the East Bay Men's Center Newsletter, and *The Periodical Lunch*, Andrew Rock publisher, Ann Arbor, Michigan, USA)

Source: U221 Unit 4 *The Changing Experience of Women* p 18.

Bibliography

Arditti, R., Duelli Klein, R. and Minden, S. *Test Tube Women*, Pandora Press, London 1984

Beechey, V. and Whitelegg, E. (eds), *Women in Britain Today*, Open University Press, Milton Keynes 1986 (see especially chapter by Doyal, L. and Elston, M. *Women, Health and Medicine*)

Bernard, J. *The Wife's Marriage*, in Evans, M. (ed), *The Woman Question*, Fontanta, London 1982

Cline, S. and Spender, D. *Reflecting Men at Twice Their Natural Size*, Fontana, London 1987

Dale, D. and Foster, P. *Feminists and State Welfare*, Routledge and Kegan Paul, London 1986

Daly, M. *Gyn/Ecology*, The Women's Press, London 1979

Ehrenreich, B. and English, D. *Complaints and Disorders: the sexual politics of sickness*, Writers and Readers, London 1973

Finch, J. and Groves, D. (eds), *A Labour of Love: Women, Work and Caring*, Routledge and Kegan Paul, London 1983

Graham, H. *Women, Health and Illness*, Social Studies Review, Vol 3 Number 1, September 1987 pp 15–20

Graham, H. *Health and Welfare*, Macmillan, London 1985

Graham, H. *Women, Health and the Family*, Wheatsheaf Books, London 1984

Graham, H. and Oakley, A. *Competing Ideologies of Reproduction; Medical and Maternal Perspectives on Pregnancy*

OPCS, *General Household Survey 1985*, HMSO, London 1987 (published annually)

Pascall, G. *Social Policy*, Tavistock, London 1986

Roberts, H. (ed), *Women, Health and Reproduction*, Routledge and Kegan Paul, London 1981 (see especially Graham, H. and Oakley, A. *Competing Ideologies of Reproduction; Medical and Maternal Perspectives on Pregnancy*)

Roberts, H. *Doing Feminist Research*, Routledge and Kegan Paul, London 1983

Showstack Sassoon, A. *From a Woman's Point of View*, Hutchinson, London 1987 (see especially Balbo, L. *Crazy Quilts* pp 45–72)

Walker, A. *Community Care: the Family, the State and Social Policy*, Blackwell and Robertson, Oxford 1982

World Bank, *World Development Report*, Oxford University Press, Oxford, published annually.

6 · Mental illness

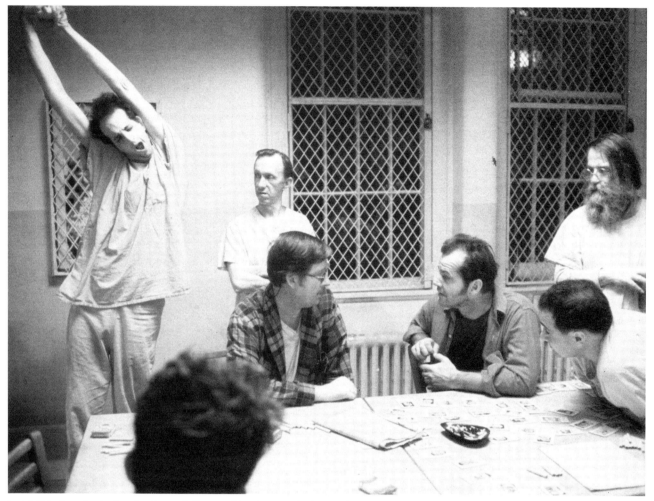

Jack Nicholson in the 'cuckoo's nest'. Do total institutions help to relieve mental illness, or to exacerbate it?

This chapter will first examine the nature of mental illness. It will then summarise the evidence about its prevalence in the UK and finally discuss alternative explanations put forward to explain its causes.

What is mental illness?

In law, mental illness is 'a state of mind which affects the person's thinking, perceiving, emotion or judgement to the extent that she or he requires care or medical treatment in her or his own interests or the interests of other persons'. Less legalistically, we can identify a continuum between mental health and mental illness. We may be at different points on this continuum at different times in our lives (though some may never get nearer to 'mad' than the gray area in the middle occupied by anxiety and depression).

Mental and emotional disorders have been classified in this way:

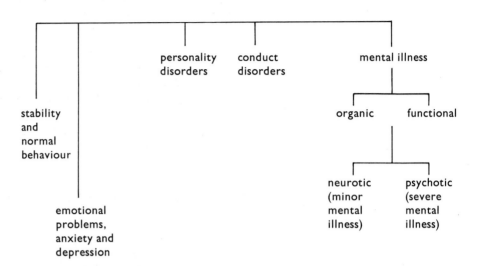

We saw in the introduction that definitions of health and illness were socially constructed. This is just as true for mental health, if not more so. Earlier in British history mental illness was seen as a sign of possession by dark forces, often as retribution for some previous evil act committed by the ill person. Even into the eighteenth and nineteenth centuries the less educated still explained mental illness in terms of devilish interference while the more educated explained it in terms of moral weakness and over-indulgence. Gradually during the last century and the early part of this century, the mentally ill came to be seen as troublesome unfortunates. Today, though, thanks to the medicalisation of mental illnesss, they are viewed as suffering from a disease analogous to physical disease. The Dean of an American University summed this change up when he said about an outbreak of witchcraft practices on campus:

> 'a couple of hundred years ago we would have burned them; twenty-five years ago I would have expelled them. Now we simply send them all to the psychiatrists'.

Today even behaviour-traits such as those associated with alcoholism are seen as evidence of disease, whereas in the past some 'fault' would have been accorded to the person involved.

☐ **Is alcoholism a 'disease' in your view?**

The statistics

In 1986 there was a total of 197,251 admissions to mental hospitals and units in England. Of these, 83,865 were male (43%) and 113, 386 were female (57%). The rate per 100,000 people in the population was 417 (total) with the rate for males 364 and females 468.

- 12.5 per cent of women and 8.3 per cent of men will need at least one stay in a psychiatric hospital during their lives.
- Informed estimates suggest that women are twice as likely to suffer from some form of mental illness as men (except as children, when males are more likely to suffer mental illness). Many of these illnesses will not lead the women to be admitted to a mental hospital, and many will be lost from view in the clinical iceberg.

- Double the number of women as men are prescribed psychotropic drugs in a year (20 per cent against 10 per cent of men).
- There are twice as many women as men admitted to mental hospitals suffering from depressive illness.

Class and ethnic origin are important too:

- Black patients are more likely to suffer compulsory admission to mental hospitals than white (though over all immigrants seem to have similar or even lower rates of admission than the indigenous population).
- Working class mothers are more likely to suffer from depression than middle class mothers.

Recent explanations of mental illness

The organic approach

This is probably the most influential approach in psychiatry. It identifies physical causes as the reason for mental illness. These may be:

- biochemical
- physiological (related to the functioning of the whole body)
- neurological (to do with the nervous system)
- anatomical
- endocrinological (concerning the glands which secrete hormones into the blood stream)
- genetic

Psychiatrists have linked certain forms of mental illness to organic causes such as epilepsy, toxins in the body (eg alcohol), nutritional disorders, brain injuries and tumours. For example, dementia is thought to be caused by disturbances in the thyroid gland in the neck which can affect the brain. In 1988, scientists at the Middlesex Hospital identified a genetic defect which they believe may be the cause of schizophrenia, which affects 500,000 people in Britain. Almost all psychiatrists would agree that *some* mental illness is caused by organic disorders; however, some say that *all* mental illness is.

Clearly, if the aetiology (cause) of the disease is physical, then the cure needs to concentrate on this, not the psychological symptoms. Treatment often involves:

- drugs (eg one of the 60 brands of tranquillisers)
- electro-convulsive treatment (ECT)
- psychosurgery—eg lobotomy, in which the tissue connecting the frontal lobe with other brain centres is severed (modern surgical methods, however, are more refined than this technique, which was mainly used in the 1950s).

The psychodynamic approach

This approach comes from psychoanalysis, which developed from the work of Sigmund Freud. He believed that we all have very strong drives which are not permitted full expression in society. These often give rise to difficulties in relationships, particularly in early life, which leave us with sets of unfulfilled desires, unresolved conflicts, suppressed fears, and so on. We are generally not conscious of these but they can affect our behaviour and in some cases give rise to symptoms of mental illness. Some psychoanalysts following this school of thought have moved away from Freud (some following other figures such as Carl Jung and Wilhelm Reich). However, the underlying principle is that adult mental illness is the product of early experiences and unconscious, suppressed, conflicts, which prevent the individual from behaving 'normally'.

The treatment for mental illness is to go through a long process of psychoanalysis in which the psychiatrist attempts to interpret the patient's conscious ideas and words in order to identify the problem or problems in the past which are the cause of the symptoms. If the patient can be encouraged to recognise the real cause and discuss it with the analyst, the contradictions will be resolved and symptoms eventually disappear.

☐ **Research the work of Jung, Reich or Freud and make a presentation to the group about it. See the bibliography for references to help.**

The behavioural approach

The behavioural approach believes that deviant behaviour (including mental illness) is the product of poor training in childhood. Children learn appropriate behaviour through a process called 'conditioning'. Desired behaviour is reinforced through rewards, while undesired behaviour is discouraged by punishment or by instilling fear (though reward has been found to be more effective than punishment). Thus some sorts of behaviour become associated with pleasure and are repeated, others with pain and are avoided. When this is not done correctly or not done enough, the person may behave oddly, or, in the jargon, 'exhibit maladaptive responses'. Also, if a certain situation or event has been followed by an unpleasant experience in the past, the two things become associated in the patient's mind. Thus seemingly harmless things may give rise to neurotic behaviour (the many phobias are thought to be the product of this sort of accidental conditioning).

☐ **Give some examples to illustrate these ideas.**

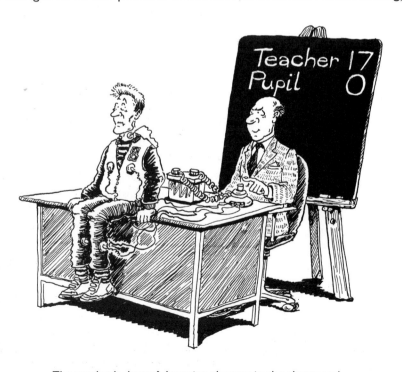

The teacher's dream? Aversion therapy in the classroom!

The treatment here is to condition the patient into new patterns of behaviour through a process of reinforcing the desired actions and (at least) discouraging the undesired ones. One way of doing this is through aversion therapy—eg administering an electric shock in the circumstances which normally lead the patient to perform the undesired behaviour. The aim is that the patient associates that situation with the unpleasant shock and so stops doing it. A more positive approach is to encourage 'adaptive responses' by rewarding appropriate behaviour with tokens which can be exchanged for privileges or luxuries.

The systemic approach

This approach sees illness as the product of the circumstances in which the patient lives, in other words as the result of a set of personal interactions in a particular context. Systemic theorists have concentrated on *the family* as an important microsystem which can lead to behaviour which is seen as symptomatic of mental illness. The mental hospital itself is another example. Dr RD Laing is the most famous psychiatrist to subscribe to this school of thought. In a series of schizophrenia cases which he treated, he shows how individuals (often girls and young women) come to exhibit bizarre behaviour as a result of oppressive family relationships. Often the mother and father treat their daughter in a way which could be deemed 'mad' itself; intercepting her letters and listening to 'phone calls, discouraging her from seeing boys (yet saying that she should), walking unannounced into her bedroom while she is undressed, treating her like a child (while insisting she should 'grow up'), and so on. In the light of this, of course, the schizophrenic behaviour begins to make sense. Yet often it is the parents who succeed in labelling their daughter: first as good, then bad, then finally mad. The same point was made by the 'mad' seventeenth century playwright Nathaniel Lee, protesting at being committed to an asylum:

> 'They called me mad, and I called them mad, and, damn them, they outvoted me'.

As the child grows up, this progression through the good–bad–mad set of labels is a common pattern of election of an individual into the category of 'mentally ill', and it is usually the family which gives the labels.

Goffman's work on mental asylums also shows how a social microsystem works. Goffman argues that far from curing people, asylums (like other 'total institutions' such as prisons) can actually cause personality disorders—'they are forcing-houses for changing persons; each is a natural experiment in what can be done to the self'. In total institutions:

- all aspects of life are conducted in the same place and under one authority;
- all activities are done in the company of a large number of other people, all are required to do the same thing together;
- all phases of the day's activities are tightly scheduled, the sequence being imposed by formal rules administered by officials;
- the enforced activities are supposedly designed to fulfill the official aims of the institution.

□ **What other examples of total institutions can you identify which fulfill these criteria?**

The word 'supposedly' is used advisedly in the last point. Goffman argues that the staff in asylums soon begin to operate on the basis of their own convenience rather than to further the interests of the patients. Patients are ignored for long periods, given sleeping tablets (so that the staff aren't troubled in the night), and are encouraged to do the staff's menial jobs 'for the exercise'. Staff themselves are in danger of becoming institutionalised and undergoing personality change. They begin to doubt which side they are on. Their response to this is to become extremely authoritarian to prove they are custodians, not inmates.

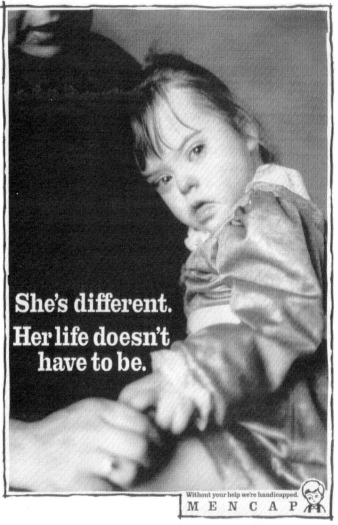

She's different. Her life doesn't have to be.

Without your help we're handicapped.
M E N C A P

Her life would be far worse if she were put in a total institution, according to Goffman.

What happens to people in total institutions is as follows. First there is a process of 'mortification', which means that the old personality of the new entrant is eradicated and his/her power of self-determination is removed. This may be done in any of the following ways:

- denying comforts like a soft bed and quietness at night
- humiliating initiation ceremonies (in some cases)
- being locked up
- restricting talk or self expression (calling people 'sir' etc)
- removing personal items like clothes, jewellery
- cutting hair

□ **Do these things occur in the examples you came up with in the exercise above?**

Having removed the old personality, the entrant to the institution is now ready to be moulded to the pattern of behaviour desired. This is achieved by:

- imposing and enforcing 'house rules'
- giving rewards and privileges for obedience
- punishing those who break the rules

The response to this by the inmate may be:

- withdrawal into an inner world. The inmate refuses to be involved in the world of the total institution. In mental hospitals this is known as 'regression', and may be seen as confirmation that the person is ill rather than as a rational response to the institution itself;
- rebellion against the staff—this is very difficult to maintain given their power, and again may be taken as a sign of mental illness;
- becoming institutionalised—seeing the total institution as a safe and desirable place to be and the outside world as threatening;
- conversion—becoming over-compliant, using the terminology of the staff, never disagreeing with them, being obsequious.

☐ **Do these also occur in your examples?**

Behaviour associated with any of these responses would, in the outside world, be considered 'mad' or at least odd. A number of factors on top of this cause the released inmate to find re-integration difficult. These include disculturation (loss or failure to acquire the habits currently required in the wider society), the stigma attatched to being an ex-inmate, the problem of once again being a small fish in a big pond rather than the reverse, and finally the fact that even on the outside there may still be some restrictions on behaviour.

The social approach

This approach stresses broader social factors than the systemic approach. While the latter is microscopic in orientation (and is associated with the interactionist school in sociology—see page 21) the social approach is macroscopic. The systemic approach looks at labelling and the medical process, particularly in total institutions. It also blames the family. According to the social approach we need to look further than behaviour within the family or mental asylums to find the causes of mental illness. Such factors as the following are thought to be to blame:

- poverty
- social isolation caused by blocks of flats and depressing environments
- mundane, repetitive work
- overcrowding
- stressful life events; divorce, exams, births and deaths etc
- sexual inequality and limiting gender roles
- consumerism
- unemployment
- instrumental relationships based on rigid hierarchies
- the stresses and strains that all this engenders

This approach helps to explain the social class and gender inequalities in mental as well as physical health. It takes the study and the treatment of mental illness out of the hands of psychiatrists and into those of sociologists. It regards as completely misconceived a systemic approach to the mentally ill which seems to say: 'our attempts to cure them have only resulted in harm—let's allow the community to try to help them'. The result is decarceration—ejecting the mentally ill from the total institutions criticised by Goffman and others. However, ejecting people into the social context which caused their illness in the first place is no way to cure it. Similarly blaming the family, as Laing does in some of his work, fails to recognise the initial causes of the family's 'mad' behaviour.

The answer, according to those who subscribe to this perspective, lies in group therapy and the establishment of therapeutic communities. We should try to set up cohesive groups of those with problems, which should give mutual support and a degree of protection from the problems listed above.

The view that mental illness is a myth

Some psychiatrists think that most mental illness is not really illness at all in the medical sense. Thomas Szasz, for example, believes that mental illness does not exist at all. Labels such as agoraphobia, hysteria, obsessive-compulsive neurosis, depression, paranoia and so on are attached to people as though they are things that *happened* to them (like catching a cold). This is nothing more than a convenient means to deal with socially disruptive problems. What medicine is saying in such cases is (for example) 'people *shouldn't* be afraid of open spaces, therefore agoraphobics are ill and need treatment to normalise them'.

> 'I hold that mental illness is a metaphorical disease; that, in other words, bodily illness stands in the same relation to mental illness as a defective television receiver stands to an objectionable television programme'. (Szasz, *The Myth of Mental Illness*, p 11)

There is really no difference in our treatment of the mentally ill and the old Soviet practice of locking dissidents up in mental hospitals—only mad people question the Soviet social and economic system. Both are nothing more than social control.

- A patient, Mrs A, is referred to a psychiatrist because she has a compulsion to wash her hands constantly. She says that the air and physical surfaces are polluted with germs and she is terrified of becoming ill through contact with them. She even blows the air in front of her mouth away constantly. She shows classic symptoms of an obsessional neurosis. How would each of the above perspectives interpret these symptoms, and how would they treat this illness?

- **ESSAY**

  How far are sociological explanations of mental illness different from, and critical of, medical ones?

- **Having read the various explanations of the causes of mental illness, and done some further reading, (see the bibliography of this chapter), complete the following table:**

approach to mental illness	main cause	key terms	best cure	criticisms
organic (etc)				

Bibliography

Asen, E. *Psychiatry for Beginners*, Writers and Readers, London 1986

Busfield, J. *Managing Madness*, Hutchinson, London

Croyden Smith, A. *Schizophrenia and Madness*, Unwin Hyman, London 1982

Gibbs, A. *Understanding Mental Health*, Consumers Association and Hodder and Stoughton, London 1986

Goffman, E. *Asylums*, Penguin, Harmondsworth, 1984 (first published 1961)

Laing, R. D. and Esterson, A. *Sanity, Madness and the Family*, Penguin, Harmondsworth 1974 (first published 1964)

Porter, R. *A Social History of Madness, Stories of the Insane*, Weidenfield and Nicholson, London 1987

Rycroft, C. *Reich*, Fontana, London 1971

Wollheim, R. *Freud*, Fontana, London 1971

Sedgwick, P. *Psycho-Politics*, Pluto Press, London 1982

Szasz, T. *The Myth of Mental Illness*, Paladin, St Albans 1973 (first published 1962)

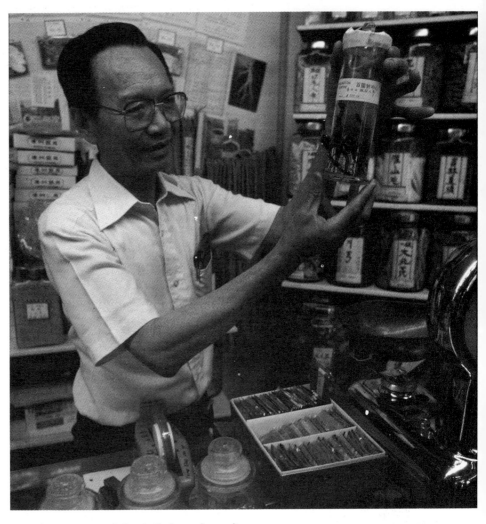

Complementary medicine in Sydney, Australia

This chapter is designed to introduce you to some of the important debates in the field of health, welfare and poverty. They can be used as a stimulus for:

- formal debates
- further research (both local and national)
- simulations
- brainstorming

The areas covered are:

- biomedicine versus alternative medicine
- the social 'problem' of ageing
- 'community care' for the mentally handicapped and others
- the role of the professions
- the effect of the welfare state on social inequality
- public versus private medicine
- drugs in society

Biomedicine versus alternative (or 'complementary') therapies

Biomedicine is the approach to medicine that is dominant in most countries in the world today. It has the following characteristics:

- It is 'scientific' (ie it only deals with observable phenomena, uses experimental methods, and seeks to establish laws to build up a body of knowledge).
- It sees the body as a physical machine, the parts of which need to be 'fixed' or even replaced when they 'go wrong'.
- Chemical (drugs) physical (surgery) and even electrical (ECT) and radiation treatments are the most successful ones.
- Biomedicine sees the world as threatening and its role being to respond to 'invasions' by viruses, bacteria, rickettsias, fungi, protozoans and the rest ('germs' in common parlance). This allopathic approach seeks to defend the body from attack by the aggressive use of 'magic bullets' of one sort or another—chemicals, radiation etc. In some cases this involves the actual use of guns.

This approach is summed up in the following quote:

'At birth you were as free of germs as the carefully sterilized instruments of the doctor who delivered you. But from the moment you took your first breath, germs entered your nose and throat; when you were first put into your cradle, germs came into contact with your skin, and from the moment you swallowed your first food, germs invaded your digestive system.'
Source: Barry, G. *Health and Wealth*, p 58

The critique of biomedicine is based on the following points:

- Some writers have noticed the similarity to elements of religion in it—the idea of sick and people being invaded by evil spirits. The allopathic approach in fact takes the wrong attitude both to the body and the environment. It doesn't ask why most of the time we can tolerate 'germs' without becoming ill, or why we do sometimes become susceptible to them. The *holistic* approach of, for example, homeopathy (see below), answers these sorts of questions (holism means they don't treat the *disease*, they treat the *patient*, taking into account all aspects of his/her life, environment, personal relationships and so on).
- Biomedicine is based on a division between mind and body—seeing the two as divided rather than forming a whole. This is referred to as 'Cartesian dualism' (from the work of the French philosopher Descartes). In biomedicine, Cartesian dualism results in the following sorts of oppositions:

Mind	versus	Body
Spirit	versus	Matter
Person	versus	Disease (medical cases)

A holistic approach rejects this dualism and sees mind and body as inseparable, a whole. One cannot be understood without an appreciation of the other.

- Biomedicine works for the current social system rather than for the ill person. For example it treats the *symptoms* of disease (headache, deviant behaviour associated with mental illness) rather than the conditions which caused them (poor environments, hazardous and stressful work).
- Biomedicine claims to have a monopoly over effective treatment; other approaches are condemned as quackery. It uses the ideology of science to back up these claims, and marshals the legislators to enforce them (legislation in 1858 set up the medical register and prevented doctors on it from cooperating with unqualified practitioners).
- Biomedicine directs the resources of the nation into the wrong areas; eg mechanical intervention such as spare-part surgery and heart operations instead of into health education and preventative medicine. This is partly because doctors want to keep medical knowledge to themselves, partly because of the bio-mechanical approach which treats the body as a machine. The NHS, under the influence of biomedicine, isn't a national *health* service but a national sickness service—a fire brigade for illness, rather than a defender of good health.
- Biomedicine does more harm than good. Doctor-caused illness ('iatrogenesis') causes much of the ill-health in Britain and other industrialised countries. 40 per cent of patients taking prescribed drugs suffer some side-effects. Many of the investigative procedures of biomedicine are painful and damaging in themselves. Many conditions, such as migraine and back-pain, are not effectively tackled by biomedical approaches, yet the attempts to do so cause problems in themselves.

☐ **Research the evidence to back up these claims. Sources that may be helpful are, for Britain, *Social Trends*, and, for abroad, some of the reference texts in the bibliography of Chapter 2.**

In reply, though, the proponents of biomedicine would argue that while there is no firm evidence of the success of other approaches, their own has been highly successful in curing many diseases, ridding the developed world of others and generally alleviating suffering. Furthermore, biomedicine *does* now recognise the importance of psychological factors in health. Biomedics are no longer Cartesian dualists.

The alternatives to biomedicine

There are as many as 135 different types of therapy which are alternatives or complementary to the biomedical approach. They range from the physical (such as osteopathy and the Alexander technique) through the psychological (such as hypnotherapy) to the paranormal (such as faith healing). Below is a list of some of the better known examples:

- homeopathy
- osteopathy
- herbalism
- acupuncture and the Chinese medical system
- naturopathy
- chiropractic
- phytotherapy

- iridology
- aromatherapy
- hydrotherapy

They have the following points in common:

- They place more emphasis than biomedicine does on preventing illness rather than curing it.
- They are 'holistic', recognising the importance of mind, body and environment. While they recognise the existence of 'germs', they realise that the person has to be susceptible for illness to result. A Professor of hygiene at Munich unversity drank a solution of cholera organisms for a bet in 1892 and nothing happened. Over forty scientists replicated the experiment. Nothing happened to any of them either!
- Their treatments are non-toxic and non-invasive, unlike those of biomedicine.
- Generally, unlike biomedicine, they do not claim to be universally effective or to have the answer to all diseases.

A survey by *Which* magazine found that two thirds of members who used alternative or complementary therapies did so after experiencing ineffective or painful biomedical intervention. The vast majority were happy with their experience, most having tried homeopathy, osteopathy or herbalism. Homeopathy is perhaps the most accepted of the complementary therapies (the Queen has a homoeopathic doctor). It holds that the symptoms presented by the sick person are not caused by the disease but by the body's action in fighting the disease off. Anything which can reinforce this will help the body. Therefore substances are given which, in a healthy person, produce the symptoms which occur when the disease is present. These are identified by a process called 'proving'—testing them on healthy people and noting the body's response. Dosages given to ill patients are tiny, and substances are heavily diluted. The dilution process ('potentisation') allegedly makes the remedy more effective; in fact the greater the dilution, the more powerful the remedy. Some evidence indicates that homeopathy is effective. Studies in the mid-1970s showed that this approach was effective in treating rheumatoid arthritis. The death rate during a cholera epidemic in the mid-nineteenth century was found to be much lower in a homeopathic hospital than in a biomedical one.

☐ **Each member of your group should research one of the complementary therapies. Make a presentation on it to the group as a whole. You might find this structure useful for your presentation:**

- **explanation**
- **background**
- **nature of the treatment**
- **comparison/contrast with biomedicine**
- **does it work?**
- **how does it work?**

The bibliography of this chapter contains some suggested reading for research and the addresses of some of the centres for these techniques in Britain.

Scientific versus holistic medicine—the arguments

Document A

'*Here's Health* magazine declares it "is committed to alternative or holistic medicine which treats people rather than disease" and that "it recognises that given the chance the body will heal itself".

But just how realistic is that claim? ... It is nonsense to say conventional medicine is not holistic. Alternative practitioners relate holism to some undiscovered "natural life force", whereas in scientific medicine holism is based on well-defined neuroendocrine pathways that link mind and body. These sensitive servo-mechanisms give us an enormous capacity for self-healing.

But what about the efficacy of alternative therapies? One recent trial of healing hypertension by laying on of hands provided intriguing evidence. Patients treated by a healer, sometimes at a distance without the patient's knowledge, showed a significant reduction in blood pressure. It sounds convincing. However, the trial also included a control group who received no treatment at all but who thought they might. They too showed a satisfactory reduction.

This study illustrates the power of the placebo effect, often adduced as evidence favouring alternative medicine. The demarcation between scientific and alternative medicine is thus a question of quality of evidence, not the treatment itself ... I recently examined one young woman who almost certainly had early breast cancer, with a 95 per cent chance of cure by limited surgery. Sadly, she was persuaded to take "holistic" treatments. If, by remote chance, it is not cancer, alternative practitioners will claim success; but if it is, and progresses, she can be blamed for not following her treatment strictly. This applies to many people with cancer. Modern medicine is their best hope.'

Source: Professor M. Baum, *Considering the Alternatives, The Observer*, 19 June 1988.

Document B

'Orthodox medicine has little time for the fringe—and vice versa. The orthodox fear the very real dangers associated with an upsurge of quacks and charlatans taking people's money and promising them the earth. The fringe fear that modern orthodox medicine is too bigoted and blinkered to be able to recognise a useful fringe therapy if it saw it ... I make no apologies for the fact that I approach patients as people who are highly complex physical and spiritual creatures. Modern medical "plumbing" has no attraction for me and I know from experience that I am not alone! The very nature of a medical care system that treats all patients with the same disease-label as though they were the same person militates against the individual treatment that people so enjoy and look for in their medical care ... A person isn't a motor-car—and is more than a collection of parts. In fact the more people know about the parts, the more questions they find. The notion, cherished by the popular press, that modern medicine is now nearer to understanding what humans are all about is completely false. Western and other therapists have huge and fundamental differences of opinion about the basic nature of the body. To many natural therapists the body's energy patterns are supremely important, yet orthodox physicians don't even admit that they exist. The functions of organs such as the liver are differently interpreted by many different therapists, and so on. We know a little about the plumbing, but by no means all there is to know'.

Source: Dr Andrew Stanway, *Alternative Medicine*, Penguin, Harmondsworth 1986 (first published 1980) pp 10–25.

□ 1 **Why is modern, *scientific*, medicine unwilling to recognise the existence of 'life forces' or 'energy patterns'?**

2 **What difference in the interpretation of the word 'holism' may exist between the doctor and the professor?**

3 **Dr Stanway's piece gives a clue to why alternative medicines are not keen on controlled experiments, in which groups of patients with the same disease are treated with alternative medicine and are compared with a control group who are not. What is the source of this reluctance?**

4 **What are your views on this debate? How would you back them up?**

□ **Before reading this section, make a list in a group of the reasons why the elderly are increasing as a proportion of the British population.**

The 'problem' of ageing

There were over nine million old age pensioners in the UK in 1988. By 2040 about 20 per cent of the population of Britain will be over 60 years old.

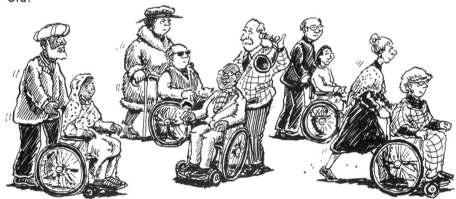

Britain in the twenty-first century?

Sociologists and policy makers tend to think of an increasingly ageing population in terms of the 'problems' they present.

The problem approach

● The old represent a burden to the rest of society. They increase the dependency ratio (ie the proportion of those who are not economically active—primarily the young and the old—compared to those who are). In 1988 half of social security spending went on old age pensioners, five million of whom relied on state benefit. The costs of all this are going to escalate, increasing the tax burden of those in work and diverting resources from investment which could improve the economy and general wealth of the country.

Table 1 Demographic factors affecting pensions

Year	Pensioners (millions)	National Insurance Contributors (millions)	Ratio of NI Contributors to Pensioners
1985	9.3	21.8	2.3
1995	9.8	21.9	2.2
2005	10.0	22.2	2.2
2015	11.1	22.4	2.0
2025	12.3	21.9	1.8
2035	13.2	21.8	1.6

□ **Summarise the trends revealed by this table. If you were in a position to advise the government on alternative responses to these trends, what would your advice be?**

Source: DHSS, *The Reform of Social Security*, Volume 2, Cmnd 9518, HMSO, London 1985, page 4.

- Old age generally sees the onset of degenerative diseases, decline in hearing and sight, loss of memory and IQ (with scores down to the level of a 10 year old by the early 60s in many cases). The incidence of long-term sickness and days of restricted activity increases sharply in old age. Over half those over 65 suffer the former, and elderly women especially suffer from the latter (48 days a year for women between 65 and 74 compared to 34 for men in the same age range).
- The decline in the birth rate, plus the increase in geographical mobility, means that many old people are alone. About 25 per cent have no children to help them. Usually the male of an elderly couple dies first, leaving the female to cope (there are twice as many women over 80 years old as men).
- About 1 per cent of people over 75 need (and get) some form of regular care (either in residential institutions or in the community).
- The Family Expenditure Survey has recorded the resources of households for over 30 years. The trend over this time has been that the resources of the elderly are declining relative to those of the non-elderly. The elderly are increasingly likely to be found among the poorest of society. Nearly two thirds of the elderly (about five million people) live in or near the margins of poverty (P. Townsend quoted in H. Graham, *Health and Welfare*, p 55).

More recently, however, the partial nature of this 'problem' approach has come to be recognised and the benefits of long life are now stressed more.

The benefits approach

- More old age pensioners have income additional to the state pension than ever before, and more have capital assets (especially houses). More than 40 per cent of the over 60s own their own home outright, half of the married couples of this age have their own car and half of the over 65s take a package holiday abroad each year.
- Better health care means that many medical problems can be eased or even cured.

- The greater spending power of the elderly means that the commercial world is catering for them to a much greater extent than in the past: this is true of the mass media, holiday companies, financial services and so on. The elderly now have great opportunities for leisure, the development of new interests, and giving more attention to old ones.

- The General Household Survey shows that 75 per cent of the over 65s are in good health. Only 3 per cent live in communal homes or hospitals and only 20 per cent suffer from senile dementia. Because of improvements in the health of elderly people death rates have declined dramatically. Between 1946 and 1985 there was a 14 per cent drop in the mortality rate of males between 65 and 74 in England and Wales while for women the equivalent figure was 30 per cent.

- While on average there *is* a decline in faculties as one ages, this is by no means an even process. *Third Age Research* found that there were many sprightly 80 year olds as well as frail and senile people in their 60s. A physically and mentally active life in adulthood can increase one's 'durability'.

- Though the elderly may make greater use of health and social services than other sections of the population, they have also made a greater contribution by paying taxes and National Insurance contributions during their lives. They are receiving what is rightfully theirs, not charity.

☐ **Illustrate this point with examples.**

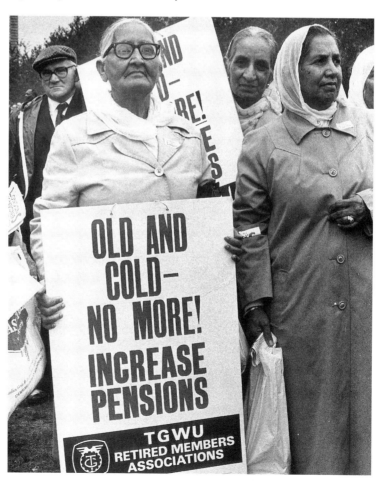

Pensioners standing up for their rights in London in the 1980s.

□ **Brainstorm the following question:**
In what areas could the elderly make the greatest contribution to society?

● The many active elderly people have a lot to contribute to society and wish to make that contribution. However, the attitudes about the elderly that are prevalent (they are dependent, have probably lost their marbles etc) make it difficult for them to be accepted.

We may now be witnessing the development of a new set of social norms in which old age is viewed positively (as it is in many non-industrial countries as well as some industrialised ones). The American Association of Retired Persons (AARP) has 29 million members and uses the slogans *Glad to be Grey* and *Grey Power*. Grey power is working in America—such a large voting block means that they can successfully put proposals for legislation to Congress. The GUMPIES (Grown Up Mature Persons) are fighting back. A British ARP has just been set up with similar goals.

□ **What are the employment characteristics most likely to determine which group an individual joins in retirement? Which sections of the population are most likely to have those characteristics?**

The truth of the matter is that there are two nations in retirement; the poor and the reasonably well off. Which category a particular person falls into largely depends upon their employment patterns during their working career.

The debate about 'community care' (or 'decarceration')

'Community care' refers to the policy of looking after the elderly, the mentally ill and physically handicapped in *society* rather than in hospitals and other institutions. It has been vigorously pursued by governments, especially in geriatric care. The number of people living permanently in hospitals or residential homes shrank by 63,000 between 1971 and 1981 (census figures). Norman Fowler, then Secretary of State for Social Services, told the House of Commons on 14 March 1986 that:

> 'we shall continue to move towards community care for the mentally handicapped and other groups of patients'.

He cited the cases of South East Thames, which by March 1987 would no longer have any children in mental handicap hospitals, and Oxford, where the 'outdated' Bradwell Grove hospital would be closed 'allowing the staff to be deployed to care for people in community units'. Despite the apparent pride the Government has in this policy it has been the subject of great debate.

'Community care' is thought to be desirable for various reasons.

● The community can act as a support for the mentally ill—social relationships have been found to be beneficial in most cases.
● The development of long acting, injectable drugs means that symptoms can be controlled on the basis of monthly treatment during a visit, rather than daily oral doses.
● Community care is cheaper than hospital care. It costs £133 to look after a mentally handicapped adult in their own home, or £119 in a local authority home with three others, compared to £255 in a mental handicap hospital. A frail elderly person looked after in their own home costs £100 per week but £295 in a NHS geriatric ward (1986 figures).
● The range of welfare provision and the number of welfare agencies now available in the community means that it is no longer necessary to shut people away.

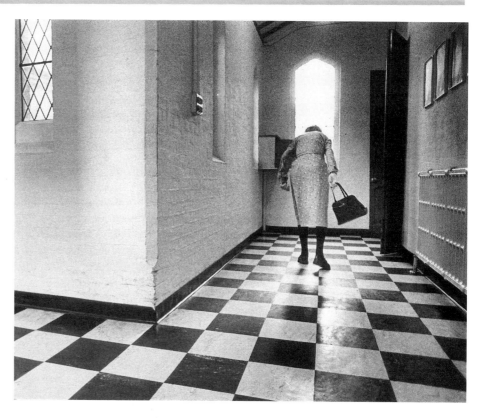

Going to church. Christmas morning at St. Lawrence's hospital for the mentally handicapped, Surrey.

- Asylums have been shown by Goffman and others to be detrimental to the mental health of patients (see page 89).

Community care sounds the perfect solution—even the name has a cosy ring to it. It is a rather ambiguous term, though. It is unclear whether it means care *in* the community (by professionals) or care *by* the community. In the 1960s the first interpretation was the dominant one. Today the latter is preferred. Of course, the concept assumes that there is a 'community' to move into. The term 'decarceration' is preferred by A. Scull. This is the opposite of incarceration (which means putting people into prison-like institutions), and stresses ejection from institutions rather than care in the community.

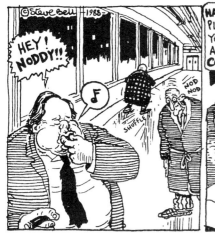
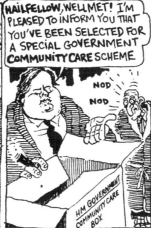
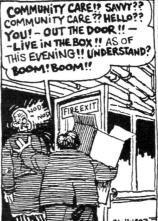
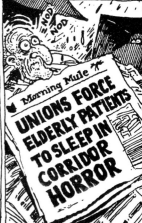

There are several problems with the policy of decarceration.

- Patients are simply thrown into the most run-down areas of cities and sea-side resorts where there is little or no community.
- Patients are given little in the way of aftercare facilities, such as the provision of employment, specialised accommodation and social support, despite the obligation placed on local authorities to provide these facilities by the 1983 Mental Health Act. They are simply dumped. So there is neither 'community', nor 'care'.
- Unscrupulous landlords specialise in providing rooms for ex-inmates. They have no medical training and little or no knowledge of patients' histories. This often results in scandalous overcrowding, poor facilities, sometimes violence, and rapid expulsion for being too troublesome. Rents, paid by the authorities, are nonetheless very high.
- Many of those 'decarcerated' are old as well as mentally ill, and have special problems and needs which makes the lack of care particularly painful for them.
- The most disturbed patients are precisely the ones who will not realise that they need help and so simply drift into obscurity until a serious problem occurs, bringing them to the attention of the police or medical services.

☐ Read (some of) E. Goffman's *Asylums* and (some of) Scull's *Decarceration* (or the extract from it in P. Trowler's *Active Sociology*.) Formulate the policy you would want implemented if you were Minister of Health.

PROJECT

☐ **Examine the map below.**

The mental hospital, (built in the middle of the last century) opposite the council estate in Factory Road has been gradually losing its patients as a result of a policy of community care and of more successful treatment and control of patients through drugs. The hospital is due to close in two years' time. Meanwhile the local Social Services Department plans to buy two empty houses in Willowtree Drive to set up a community hostel for a small number of patients currently in the hospital. This plan has been leaked to the press and residents in the area have called for a public meeting to discuss the issue and to allow them to air their views. Choose

Helmington

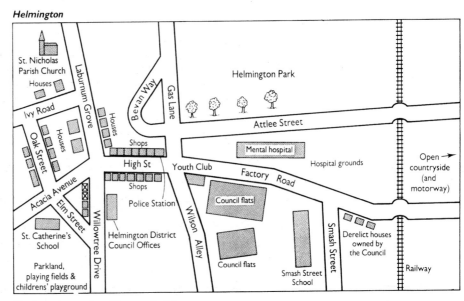

☒ = Empty houses planned for use as hostel

roles from those outlined below and spend about 15 minutes planning your arguments for the public meeting. Then hold the meeting:

Director of Social Services and staff (including **Finance Director**);

you should be prepared to put forward the advantages of the policy of community care in general, and the points in favour of a hostel in this location in particular. You are very keen to see the hospital closed for a variety of reasons.

Residents around Willowtree Drive;

you are concerned about a number of issues here. You are prepared to admit some of your worries (danger to children from the residents of the hostel etc) but are rather embarrassed about others (falling property prices etc). You don't wish to be seen to be against the interests of the mental patients and so you want to be able to make an alternative proposal rather than simply block this one.

Council tenants;

you should consider your views about the closure of the mental hospital near to your estate and give careful thought to any alternative plans that the Social Services Department might have should they meet stiff opposition to the Willowtree Drive proposal.

The Press;

should take notes on the meeting and, after it has finished, find a quiet room to rough out a headline and a brief summary of the article you would write about it for the local paper (the Helmington Gazette). Read this to the other participants after the meeting.

The Vicar of Helmington;

you should form your own view on this issue, but bear in mind the feelings of your parishioners.

The Chair of the meeting;

your role is to be impartial and to make sure that there is an orderly debate in which all sides are heard.

Councillors;

Helmington District Council is a "hung" council, ie no one political party holds overall control. Helmshire County Council, though, is Conservative controlled. Represented are district councillors from the Democrats, Conservatives and Labour, and County Councillors from the Conservatives. These should formulate their party's views on the issue (and their own, if these differ).

The debate about the role of the professions

W. J. Good cites two core characteristics of a profession:

- prolonged specialised training in a body of abstract thought;
- a collectivity or service orientation (ie working for other people).

Associated with these are ten further characteristics.

1 The profession determines its own standards of education and training.

☐ **According to these criteria, would you regard the following as professionals (and if not why not)?:** nurses, teachers, solicitors, prostitutes ('the oldest profession'), chiropodists, senior police officers, soldiers, social workers.

2   The student goes through a deeper socialisation experience than learners in other occupations.

3   Professional practice is recognised by some form of licence.

4   Licensing and admission boards are staffed by members of the profession.

5   Most legislation concerned with the profession is shaped by it.

6   There are high rewards in terms of income, power and prestige so that high calibre students can be attracted.

7   The practitioner is relatively free of evaluation and control by lay people.

8   The norms of practice enforced by the profession are more stringent than legal controls.

9   Members are more strongly identified and affiliated with the profession than is usual in other occupations.

10 Members do not normally leave the profession and are usually happy to be in it.

For functionalist sociologists, as for many people in general, the higher professions such as doctors are virtually beyond reproach. Professionals are seen as selfless individuals working for the good of the community, often making great personal sacrifices. They need to be of the highest intelligence and skill, have to undergo years of training, and in their early careers earn very little. High levels of reward later, then, are necessary to attract, retain and motivate the best people into the professions.

Against this altruitistic view of the professionals, though, the following charges have been levelled:

● There is very little control over them. Professional bodies (such as the General Medical Council) are charged with supervising the profession. But, being composed of members of that profession themselves, they usually whitewash or ignore cases of incompetence etc. Final sanctions, like striking a doctor off the medical register, are used only rarely and then more often for sexual misconduct than gross incompetence.

● They use the argument of 'professional expertise' as a smokescreen for practices which in other areas would not be permitted, for example maintaining the monopoly over the provision of particular goods or services, and price fixing. Examples are numerous; the restriction on advertising the services of solicitors and opticians was only recently lifted. The professionals claimed that the prohibition maintained the level of the service by preventing over-concentration on price. Actually it was to maintain profits by preventing 'harmful' competition between members of the same profession.

● They artificially restrict numbers entering the profession in order to increase demand for those already in it and therefore raise the fees they can charge for their services. This means that the community suffers unnecessary shortages of professionals.

● They do a bad job. Doctors' drug prescriptions cause bad side effects and sometimes dependency. Their diagnostic tests do more harm than good in many cases. Women in particular suffer at their hands. Many iatrogenic (doctor-caused) diseases affect women only, for example those stemming from using contraceptive pills and devices, and from hysterectomies. Doctors medicalise pregnancy and birth, taking control away from women and treating them merely as 'cases'. Doctors and social workers can and do abuse their power, as occurred in the Cleveland child abuse scandal of 1987 (see the British Humanities Index for references to newspaper accounts of this). Generally the professionalisation of medicine means that responsibility for our health and our lives is taken from our hands and put in those of doctors, nurses, psychiatrists, social workers and the rest. This alienates us from our own existence.

The Welfare State and inequality

Many proponents of the Welfare State argue that its aim is more than the elimination of the 'five giants' identified by Beveridge. It is also there to bring about greater equality within British society. This

The best off contribute most money towards the Welfare State

Arguments in favour	Arguments against
Income tax is progressive—ie the better off have to pay 60 per cent while the lower earners pay only 25 per cent.	Yes, it is progressive, but far less so than in the past. The better off had to pay well over the basic rate on much of their income (up to 83 per cent). Now they pay only 60 per cent maximum and 25 per cent on much of their income.
The lower earners have a fairly high proportion of tax-free income (ie the tax threshold is quite high). Higher earners pay tax on a higher proportion of their income.	The tax threshold has been falling for years, relative to incomes, bringing even quite poor people into the tax net and increasing the number of tax payers.
National Insurance contributions are based on a percentage of salary, so that the poor pay less as their incomes are lower. Insurance-based *benefits*, though, are frequently at a fixed level.	There is an upper limit of earning beyond which National Insurance contributions are not deducted. So, while the poorest pay NI on most of their income, the better off will escape it on a substantial part of theirs. Also NI is not payable on income such as rent, interest from savings accounts and dividends from shares.
VAT is paid at 15 per cent on goods. However, many basic necessities are VAT free, thus helping the poor who spend much of their income on these things.	Different rates of VAT (higher on luxury goods) have been abolished and VAT has been levied on an increasingly wide range of products. The poorest pay more VAT as a proportion of income because they spend most of their income on goods while the rich can save much of theirs. Tax on goods, like VAT, is *regressive*—it hits the poorest hardest.
Rates, because they are higher for those with bigger and more luxurious homes, are a progressive form of taxation.	Poll tax will soon replace rates and this is heavily regressive—being based on people rather than property. A large family living in a cramped house will pay far more than an affluent couple living in a large house.
Capital is taxed as well as income (eg by Capital Transfer Tax) and this form of tax is likely to be paid only by the better off.	True, but less than 2 per cent of Government income is derived from this source, compared to about 25 per cent from income tax and 12.5 per cent from VAT. The non-payment of capital tax by the poor is outweighed by their greater payment of excise duty on alcohol and tobacco, both in real terms and as a proportion of their income.

☐ **Students should divide into two groups. One is led by the Minister of Health in a radical new British Government that wishes to see fundamental changes in the medical profession. Senior civil servants are there to help him/her formulate the proposals. Before the meeting the members should do some research on the present problems with the medical profession, to determine precisely what needs to be put right. Refer to: Illich, I. *Medical Nemesis* and Graham, H. and Oakley, A. *Ideologies of Reproduction*.**

The second group represents the BMA. They should develop all the arguments and evidence they can to try to persuade the Minister and his/her advisers that change would be a bad thing. Try to predict the arguments that will be raised in the meeting and prepare counter arguments to them, as well as being ready to put your own side of the case. Decide what threats you can make if the Minister is intransigent.

When both sides are ready, hold the meeting. The Minister, advised by the civil servants, must make a decision at the end of it. S/he should try to be as open-minded as possible and make a realistic assessment of the possible consequences of any decision.

The worst off receive most benefits and services from the Welfare State

Arguments in favour	Arguments against
The poor benefit most from means-tested benefits such as income support because only they are eligible for them.	In terms of government spending most money goes on universal benefits—ie ones received by everybody in a certain category regardless of income. These include pensions, child benefit, invalidity benefit, unemployment and sickness benefit. Also the better off will gain more from the 'fiscal social security' of tax relief on private pensions following the 1986 Social Security Act, as they will be most likely to take out such pension plans.
The poor benefit most from state health and education service because the better off can opt out into the private system.	Many people never go private, and those who do still take advantage of many state services. Furthermore, the better off are more likely to send their children to higher education (which is subsidised by the state), and the state schools which their children do attend are likely to be better funded and more successful than those in deprived areas.
The poor are the only ones likely to take advantage of council housing—thus they benefit from its subsidies.	Council housing now has to pay its own way and better off tenants are buying their council houses, leaving only low quality housing for those who remain. Home owners get tax relief on mortgages regardless of their income (more 'fiscal social security') and also benefit from house price rises.
The poor are sicker than the better off (see p. 60), therefore they will make most use of health services. Inhabitants of inner-city areas, especially in London, have good access to excellent hospitals.	The better off generally have greater access to better facilities of all sorts and make proportionately greater use of them relative to their level of health.
The poor make greater use of public transport and so benefit from state subsidy of it.	Actually the better off benefit most from transport subsidies—especially rail (eg London commuters) and from road building and maintenance programmes. The better off get hidden subsidies in the form of company cars, and expense accounts as well as company pensions, membership of private health schemes and other perks. This 'occupational welfare' is subsidised by the state through tax relief to companies that provide it.

Percentage increase in earnings after tax and nation
insurance 1979-86. (Married man with non-working wife and tv
children).

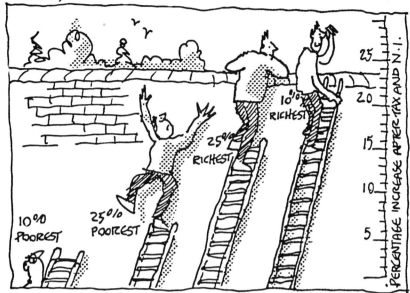

Change in income tax and national insurance
contributions as a percentage of gross income (1978-79 to 1986-87)

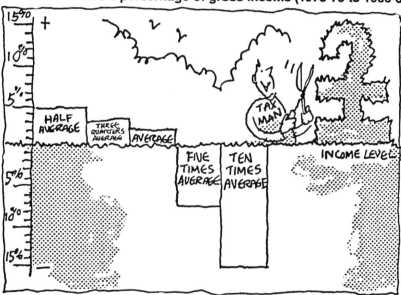

Source: *New Society*, 'The Decade of Inequality', 6 February 1987.

'strategy of equality' (as Tawney called it) involves funding services and benefits for the worse off by taxing the better off—the Robin Hood welfare state. On the face of it this would appear to be happening; richer people 'obviously' pay more into the Welfare State and poorer people equally obviously get more out. But do they? In order to see whether this is really the case we need to examine closely the two central propositions in the idea of the strategy of equality:

- the best off contribute most money towards the Welfare State;
- the worst off receive most benefits and services from it.

Trying to assess the overall effect of taxation to determine whether it is progressive, regressive or proportional is quite difficult. Income tax and National Insurance combined are progressive until the middle levels of income, then they are proportional. Thus the middle fifth of income

☐ **Why has the Conservative's tax policy had the result of being less redistributive? (Look again at the arguments of the New Right, pp 22–24.)**

earners pay as much (as a proportion of their income) as the highest two fifths, but more than the lowest two fifths of income earners.

Commodity taxes such as VAT and excise duty are very regressive, as is poll tax. Capital tax, on the other hand is progressive. Overall, the evidence indicates that while the very poorest pay less tax than everybody else, those above the very lowest levels of income will pay the same amount of tax as a proportion of income, regardless of the level of that income. So, the Robin Hood state takes from the rich, the comfortable and the 'nearly poor' to the same degree. But does the money go to the 'really poor'?

We are now in a position to assess the overall effect of the welfare benefit system. It certainly helps to reduce poverty considerably, but it does not seem to do much in terms of bringing about greater equality. Julian LeGrand argues:

> 'of all current expenditure on social services it can be estimated that only about one fifth is directed primarily at the poor. All the rest is either distributed equally or towards the better off'.

Table 2 demonstrates the effect of taxes and benefits on inequality.

Table 2 The effects of taxes and benefits on inequality, 1982, (% share of total income)

Group	Original income	Gross income	Disposable income	Final income
Top fifth	47%	41%	40%	39%
Next fifth	27%	25%	24%	24%
Middle fifth	18%	18%	18%	18%
Next fifth	7%	11%	12%	12%
Bottom fifth	0.4%	5.7%	6.8%	6.9%

Source: LeGrand, Open University unit, p 19.

Original income = before taxes or state subsidies
Gross income = original income plus income subsidies such as Income Support
Disposable income = gross income less income tax
Final income = disposable income plus the value of all subsidies like public transport less the cost of commodity taxes like VAT

□ **What were the shares of original income of the top and bottom 40 per cent of the population in 1982?**

What was the effect of taxes and benefits on inequality in 1982?

□ **ESSAY**

> **'Social services do little to equalise the distribution of rewards flowing from the institutions of market, private property and inheritance' (R. Mishra, *Society and Social Policy*).**

a) **What are the arguments in support of this statement? (10 marks)**
b) **How far is it true? (15 marks)**

Public versus private medicine

The pros and cons of private medicine

Cons	Pros
Private patients see the same consultants as NHS ones—they don't get improved treatment	Private medicine gives the individual choice—it is patient-centred, not run on bureaucratic lines
Private hospitals have a limited range of facilities and few full time staff (about 74 per cent do not have a resident doctor)	Some sorts of treatment are only available under private medicine—eg most cosmetic surgery
Private hospitals find it difficult to recruit full-time doctors because they have not been accredited for training purposes. High-quality staff, in particular, are difficult to attract	Private patients in hospital get privacy and one-to-one treatment
Staff are expensively trained by the NHS and then lost to the private sector—this is a drain on state resources	Medics and paramedical staff can increase their earnings through private practice
Some consultants may artificially create NHS waiting lists in order to attract more patients into private practice	The NHS benefits from income from pay beds, donations of equipment by private medicine to be used both for NHS and private patients, and from reduced waiting lists resulting from patients going private rather than joining NHS lists
Doctors spending time on private patients means they have less time for NHS ones, thus lengthening NHS waiting times	Some consultants invest in private hospitals and benefit from the income they generate
NHS staff have an additional work load as a result of doctors being absent on private medical business	There are increasing numbers of private facilities for geriatric and other chronic medical cases
Pay beds—ones rented out to the private sector by the NHS—often cost more to service than the money they raise, especially when private patients in them require treatment which is heavily capital or labour intensive	Consultants treat private patients better (eg they are more likely to be on time for appointments)
Private medicine can lead to 'medical inflation', ie doctors providing unnecessary treatment for profit motives	There are shorter waiting lists in private practice—patients can get treatment quickly
Medical resources are even more concentrated in the affluent parts of the country because private medicine is attracted there	Competition between private companies improves the service all round
Administrative costs are higher because of the complicated and replicated fee and payment structure and advertising costs	Some private hospitals do train nurses
Private medicine in general is good at 'cure' not 'care' (ie acute rather than chronic medicine)	Private medicine generates profit and attracts foreigners to this country for paid treatment, thus adding to the national wealth
There are ethical problems if doctors are shareholders in private hospitals	Private pharmaceutical companies generate new drugs and techniques very successfully, private medical care organisations can be similarly innovative.
Generally, the state should take responsibility for the health of people—cheque-book medicine only increases social divides	

☐ **Some of the points in the left and right columns can be said to answer each other. Re-arrange the columns to match the points which address the same issue.**

What ethical problems might result from a doctor being a shareholder in a private hospital?

There are basically three types of private medicine:

- fee for service
- private insurance cover
- premiums to medical organisations

☐ **Devise a questionnaire designed to elicit people's attitudes about private medicine. If possible conduct the survey.**

Agencies providing private medicine range from charitable organisations (for example church-run hospitals) to provident organisations (eg BUPA, which are theoretically non-profit making but in fact have subsidiaries which are profit-oriented), to 'for profit' organisations such as American Medical International.

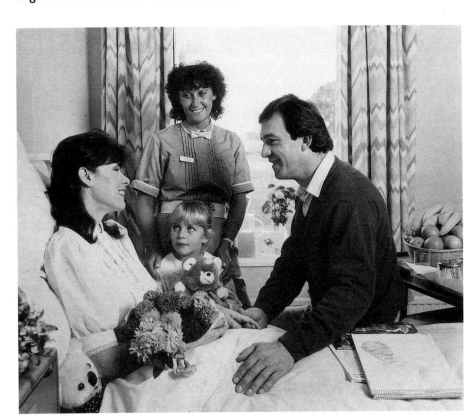

☐ **Individually, write a paragraph commenting on this photograph. If you are familiar with semiological analysis, try applying that approach. When you have done this, compare your comments with those of the other people in the group you are studying with.**

BUPA advertises the benefits of its private medicine schemes.

Drugs and society

☐ **Before beginning this section, complete the following sentences on your own. Then compare and discuss what you have written with other group members:**

1 **When thinking about drugs I think about ...**
2 **Drug users tend to be ...**
3 **The media's portrayal of drug use is ...**
4 **People use drugs because ...**
5 **The effects of drugs are ...**
6 **The drug we need to worry most about is ...**
7 **We can find drug users easily if we go to ...**

This section will look at common conceptions about drugs that exist in society and then go on to question them.

Common conceptions about drugs

□ **For what reasons might that be an inaccurate description of the average heroin user?**

- Drug users have particular characteristics. For example the typical heroin user, as identified by studies of those who come to the attention of doctors, police or the social services, is likely to fit the following description:

  male
  in his late teens or early twenties (the average age is dropping)
  single
  product of a single parent family or separated from both parents
  poorly educated
  unemployed or in casual labour
  unable to give up the drug
  suffers from illnesses associated with drug use
  has a criminal record unrelated to drug use
  is on prescribed drugs to control and limit his use of heroin

- Solvent abusers ('glue sniffers') on the other hand tend to be:

  between 11 and 16 years
  male
  short-term users
  concentrated in one locality

- Cocaine users are likely to be older and more affluent than either of these.
- Particular areas of the country have a drug problem. For example Liverpool has become known as 'Smack City' in the tabloids and Merseyside in general is viewed as having a drugs problem.
- 'Soft' drug use leads on to 'hard' drugs. The addict is likely to climb a drugs ladder which looks like this:

  ↑ Opiates, including heroin ('smack', 'junk')
  LSD ('acid')
  mixed drugs (eg 'ecstasy' = amphetamines + LSD)
  barbiturates ('sleepers', 'downers')
  amphetamines ('pep-pills', 'speed', 'uppers')
  cannabis ('grass', 'pot', 'hash')
  hallucinogenics ('magic mushrooms')
  solvents ('glue sniffing')

- Once on this ladder of bad drugs the user becomes progressively 'hooked'—physically addicted to the effects of the drug. Coming off them will require a very unpleasant and prolonged period of adjustment involving severe physical symptoms.
- Climbing the ladder is expensive. Eventually the user will have to turn to crime to fund the habit. Violent crime is made more likely by the loss of inhibitions caused by drug use.
- There are 'good drugs' and 'bad drugs'. 'Good' ones are fairly harmless, even beneficial. They include tobacco, caffeine and medically prescribed drugs such as Librium and Valium. Alcohol is also a 'good drug' (or not even thought of as a drug at all), though it is potentially harmful if taken by the wrong kind of people— particularly 'lager louts'.

- What is needed is strong will-power, to resist drugs in the first place or, later, to get off the ladder as soon as possible. The user needs to JUST SAY NO (the catchphrase of a campaign against drug use launched by Nancy Reagan during her husband's US presidency). Individual free will, not economic or social circumstances, are to blame. There are strong connections here with the 'culture of poverty' theory—people can and should choose to reject that culture.
- The reason why people become drug takers in the first place (despite the obvious drawbacks) is that they are persuaded by drug pushers who are concerned purely with profit. It is these people to whom one should 'just say no'.

☐ **Generally, how do you respond to this view of drugs and drug users?**

Problems with this view

- Users who come to the attention of the official agencies are not typical. The middle class and those who have never needed or wanted to refer themselves to agencies are under-represented in the studies and statistics.
- Similarly, areas of the country with large numbers of 'drug-prone types' will be targeted in the press as problem-centres. Academic studies will then concentrate on them, giving them further prominence. In fact virtually everyone uses drugs of some sort, including alcohol, caffeine and 'medical drugs'. Every society in history, with the exception of two groups of indigenous Alaskans, has had a drug or drugs as a central part of its culture. Britain's is alcohol, in many muslim countries it is hashish, and in Mexico it was hallucinogens found in cacti.
- Evidence shows that many people experiment with drugs and never use them again. Even persistent drug users go through periods of heavy and light use. There is little hard evidence on the 'progression up the ladder' hypothesis. Instead there are 'experimental users' (in the majority) who experiment and stop, 'recreational users' who use one type of drug occasionally and without problems, and 'problem users' (in the minority) who are dependent and for whom, or for those around them, their drug-taking is causing a problem.
- So called 'good drugs' can be more harmful than 'bad drugs'. Smoking causes about 100,000 premature deaths every year. Persistent heavy drinking causes brain cell and liver damage. In 1986 there were 18,000 hospital admissions for alcohol-related disorders, not to mention the hundreds of thousands of alcohol-related crimes. 'Medical' drugs such as the benzodiazapines Librium, Valium and Mogadon (commonly known as tranquillisers and/or sleeping pills) cause physical and psychological dependence and symptoms such as depression, tiredness, difficulty in concentration, agoraphobia and headaches. About half a million people have suffered at least a mild dependence on them, and around three and a half million people have taken tranquillisers 'well into the period when they may have lost their useful effect, and become potentially dangerous', according to one survey. Most of those prescribed benzodiazapines are women (four women to each man).

- The paradox is, however, as one expert states, that "bad" drugs such as heroin, cocaine and cannabis produce no such tissue damage, and problems arising from their use stem mainly from their illegal status and subsequent impurity, contamination and septic use' (Robertson p 20).

  Another author (Jock Young) uses the term 'The Law of Inverse Effect' to describe the relationship between our attitudes to a drug and the damage it does.

☐ **Brainstorm the following questions in small groups:**

1 **Why is so much negative attention paid by the media and the Government to the drugs which damage the smallest number of people, while so little is paid to the most damaging ones; alcohol and tobacco?**
2 **Why are drugs like cannabis illegal when they do so little damage, yet tobacco and alcohol are legal and freely available (with only loosely enforced rules regarding age limits)?**

In larger groups, collate and discuss your ideas.

Educationalists, and those in positions of responsibility, are very concerned about the use of 'bad drugs' by the young, but a *New Society* survey conducted in 1986 showed that the young are far more likely to use the 'good drugs'.

Table 3: Drug use by age and sex

	Total	Male	Female	Under 14	14–16	17–19	Over 19
Total in sample	2,417	725	1,692	235	977	992	213
Which of the following have you tried? (figures are given in percentages)							
Cigarettes	65	64	65	60	67	63	69
Cannabis	17	24	14	7	12	19	37
Heroin	2	3	1	3	1	1	5
Solvents	6	10	4	8	6	6	6
Alcohol	89	90	88	85	88	92	82
Not stated	7	6	8	10	8	6	10
Which of the following drugs do you think is the most dangerous in terms of the effect it has? (figures are given in percentages)							
Cigarettes	21	22	20	14	20	22	25
Cannabis	2	2	1	3	1	2	1
Heroin	56	55	57	71	61	52	40
Solvents	5	4	5	3	5	5	3
Alcohol	16	16	16	8	12	18	29
Not stated	1	1	1	1	1	1	2

Source: M. Williams, *The Thatcher Generation*, New Society, 21 February 1986

☐ 1 **What conclusions can be drawn from these results?**
2 **Why should these conclusions be treated cautiously?**

- Evidence now points to the fact that 'addiction' is the wrong word to use as it implies physical need for a substance. Specialists in the field now prefer to use the word dependence. This means a psychological and/or physical compulsion to take a drug in order to experience its effects or to avoid the discomfort of its absence. Alcohol and the opiates (eg opium, morphine, methadone) create both physical and psychological compulsions. Current research suggests that amphetamines, cocaine, cannabis and the hallucinogens (such as LSD) create a psychological compulsion only (though this is not certain).

- Users of prescribed drugs are by definition 'criminals'. Also, some drug users will be criminals in just the same way that some tobacco smokers are; their criminality is unrelated to their drug use. Furthermore, if we assume that drug users are more likely to come from the poorer section of the community (though this is not necessarily the case, as we saw above), then we would expect them to have a higher rate of recorded crime anyway, as this section of society are more criminal (at least according to official statistics) than the rest. The question is, does drug use result in a subsequently greater chance of criminal activity in the individual than would otherwise be the case? The answer is that we don't really know, and even if we did the reasons would not be clear. The reasons could be the need for money, and decreased inhibitions, or be more complex than this.

  Jock Young argues in *The Role of the Police as Amplifiers of Deviancy* that the police's pursuit of drug-takers marginalises them from ordinary society, forcing them into a closed world, and turning them into criminals by making life difficult for them in the 'straight' world. This process illustrates well the point the interactionist Howard Becker was making when he wrote: 'social groups create deviance by making the rules whose infraction constitutes deviance'. In other words, (in this case), if proscribed drugs were legalised there would be no greater crime associated with them than with (for example) tobacco.

- Many experts in the field see drug-taking not as sign of individual weakness in not being able to 'say no', but as a product of particular social and economic circumstances. Like alcohol, drugs such as opium and methadone give a sense of well-being and release from current problems. The fit person with good prospects may not need this but the person who was a failure at school, has limited prospects and lives in a deprived area will find drugs a convenient escape route. This view of drug use and users accords more with the poverty trap approach of the social democrats than with the culture of poverty thesis of the New Right.

- Jock Young, in the study referred to above, argues that while there *are* pushers now, these are the product of the law enforcement activities of the police, which restricted the supply of drugs and hence pushed their prices up. Seeing a highly profitable market develop, the criminal world moved into the drugs trade, resulting in the appearance on the scene of the 'pusher'. Robertson argues in the case of heroin that:

  'Most [dealers of heroin] are users themselves and finance their own use this way rather than indulging in other criminal activities ... The stereotype of pushers who hang around street corners or outside schools and tempt newcomers to use drugs is equally fallacious and likely, if it did occur, to increase the chances of being arrested rather than increase profits'. (p 46)

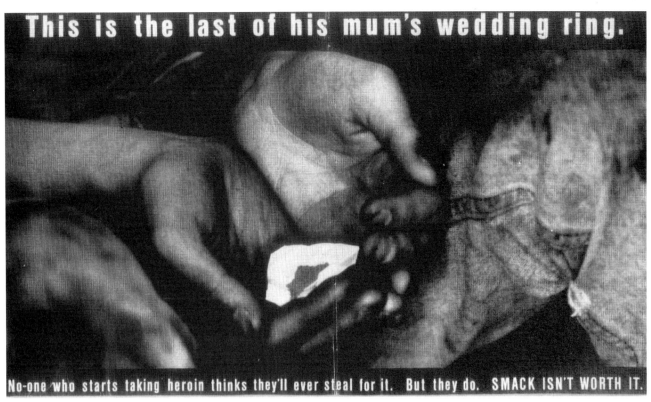

Aiming to change people's behaviour—the DSS tries to limit heroine use.

☐ In the light of the above information, create ideas for a government health warning poster like the heroin one above but for cigarettes and/or whisky.

☐ A meeting has been called by the Director of a college in your area to discuss the issue of drug abuse by young people at the college and in the area generally. The meeting must:

● write a policy statement for the college—ie a statement of the 'position' of the college on drugs. It may be adopted by the County Council as a whole;
● incorporate in it a set of guidelines for staff employed by the Council on how to deal with any drug abuse that comes to their attention (eg among students at the college).

The meeting is chaired by the Director and it comprises:

Local business people (from the college's Governing Body)
The community policeman/woman
Social and youth workers employed by the County
Lecturers at the college
A specialist running a hostel for drug abusers trying to come off them
A doctor
An education adviser from County Hall
The lecturer in charge of running the pastoral care system in the college
Parents (from the college's Governing Body)

Choose your roles and spend about ten minutes working out your position on the issue in detail (make notes if you need to). At the end of that time the meeting should be convened by the Director. From then on act in role. It is the Director's responsibility, as Chair, to ensure that the aims of the meeting are achieved within the time allocated.

☐ **The following three sets of columns list types of drug, their effects and the long term risks associated with them. However they have been jumbled up! Your task is to match the boxes in the three columns with each other. Finally you should say whether that drug is: legal, illegal, illegal to sell to anyone under a certain age, illegal for someone under a certain age to buy or use, legal unless made into a preparation, illegal unless prescribed, or legal but only available on prescription. Answers are in the bibliography.**

DRUG	EFFECTS AND MANNER OF USE	RISK
1 SOLVENTS (eg glue, lighter fuel)	It makes you feel warm and drowsy, kills pain. It can cause constipation and a feeling of sickness. Under its influence it is difficult to concentrate and slows your reactions, it can be smoked, sniffed or injected and its effects can last for several hours.	Users need to take larger and larger doses to get the same effect. There is a risk of paranoia which can develop into serious mental illness. Neglect of the dietary and sleep needs of the body under the influence of the drug can lead to illness. It is difficult to break the habit and high doses can damage the heart.
2 AMPHETAMINES ("speed", "uppers")	It relaxes you, increases the pulse rate and the blood pressure while reducing the appetite. It produces carbon monoxide which is absorbed by the lungs. Its effects can last for some hours, It is smoked or chewed.	People can do dangerous things while hallucinating, including accidentally killing themselves. It can also lead to mental illness. Deaths from overdose are unknown, though, and physical addiction seems not to occur.
3 LSD ("acid")	It is absorbed into the bloodsteam. Small amounts make you friendly, relaxed and talkative, large amounts make speech blurred, vision diminished, concentration reduced and reactions slowed. It is swallowed.	The main risk is from accidental death or injury while affected, choking on vomit following unconsciousness and from freezing the tubes in the lungs as a result of squirting the very cold gas into the mouth. It can result in brain damage in the long term.
4 CAFFEINE (eg coffee)	It makes you feel strong and confident, reduces the appetite and enables you to work harder. You feel tired and depressed after it has worn off, though (which is not very long after taking it). It is sniffed up the nose or injected in to the bloodstream.	This can cause damage to the heart, liver, stomach and brain. Accidents and violence resulting from the diminished control over one's actions is the major cause of the many deaths and injuries related to this drug. Overdose or choking on vomit following unconsciousness are also risks. Occasional heavy use can result in headaches, sickness and irritability the following day.
5 BARBITURATES (eg sleeping pills)	It affects people in different ways, and some claim to be not affected by it. Small amounts can result in a feeling of well-being, talkativeness and giggling, larger amounts in forgetfulness and withdrawal. These effects usually subside after an hour or so. It is usually smoked (mixed with tobacco) or eaten.	Regular use can result in cancer, blood clots, heart disease, strokes, poor circulation and ulcers. Withdrawal from regular use can result in irritability, headaches and depression.

6 TRANQUILLISERS ("downers", eg Librium and Valium)

You may become light-headed, feel very confident and even see and hear things with greater clarity. Hallucinations are possible and you may feel sick and get stomach ache. Effects can last for as much as a day, It is usually drunk as a tea or eaten, sometimes cooked.

Overdose can be fatal and there is a risk of infection from AIDS and other diseases through needle sharing. People become dependent quickly and withdrawal is painful, leading to shakes, sweating, stomach cramps and so on. Addiction to the drug can lead to dangerous activities to obtain it.

7 CANNABIS ("grass", "pot")

You feel relaxed and will go to sleep with larger doses (and this drug is often used for this). After taking several of these the user loses control of speech and other faculties. The effect can last for up to six hours and the drug is usually taken in pill form (though it can be injected as a diluted powder).

Deaths are rare, though if it is injected there is a risk of infection from shared needles. There seems to be a high risk of physical dependence, though if it is given up there are few long-term consequences.

8 'MAGIC' MUSHROOMS

It calms you down and makes you feel drowsy. It makes you feel less anxious and stressed, and is often used specifically for this. It lasts for up to six hours and is usually taken in pill form (though it can be injected as a diluted powder).

Few serious consequences, though some people suffer a deterioration in memory and some may become temporarily mentally disturbed. There can be a risk of lung damage when smoked and it is dangerous to drive under its influence.

9 COCAINE ("coke", "snow")

It keeps you awake and aids concentration. A lot can inceease the heart rate and make you shaky as well as increasing the number of times you urinate. Its effects can last for a number of hours and it is usually drunk.

The biggest risk is in picking the wrong sort as some varieties are poisonous. There are no withdrawal symptoms and apparently no long-term damage, though high doses can cause temporary sickness and stomach pain.

10 HEROIN-LIKE DRUGS ("smack", "H" etc)

It makes you energetic and alert though it can increase anxiety levels. One dose can last for two days and when it has worn off you feel tired, depressed and hungry very often. It is usually taken as tablets, though can be injected or sniffed.

Accidents can result from loss of body control. Large doses can cause loss of consciousness, breathing problems and death (this drug is sometimes used as a method of suicide). Mixing with alcohol can be very dangerous.

11 TOBACCO

It can have quite powerful effects on your senses and perceptions, perhaps causing hallucinations. While under its influence you are unable to do much, and might be very excited or – if it's a "bad trip" – terrified.

Peptic ulcer, cancer and heart disease are thought to be made more likely by the use of this drug in large quantities (say, more than 8 cups a day). Physical dependence can occur and withdrawal leads to headaches, irritability and drowsiness.

12 ALCOHOL

It goes directly to the brain and makes you feel light-headed. Its effect is quite short lived (less than an hour usually) and may leave you with a hangover (though it can also be fatal). It is always sniffed through the nose, sometimes from inside a plastic bag over the head.

People using this drug need more and more to get the same effect and eventually feel that they cannot live normally without it. Withdrawal can cause anxiety, sickness and headaches, even fits (after high doses).

Bibliography

Barry, G. *et al*, (eds), *Health and Wealth*, Macdonald, London 1965

Breckon, W. *Your Everyday Drugs*, BBC, London 1978

Clover, A. *Homeopathy: A Patient's Guide*, Thorsons Publishers, Wellingborough 1984

Dingwall, R. and Lewis, P. (eds), *The Sociology of the Professions: Lawyers, Doctors and Others*, Macmillan, London 1983

Glennerster, H. *The Future of the Welfare State*, Heinemann, London 1983—see especially the article by LeGrand

Goffman, E. *Asylums*, Penguin, Harmondsworth, 1984 (first published 1961)

Graham, H. and Oakley, A. *Ideologies of Reproduction*, in Roberts, H. (ed), *Women, Health and Reproduction*, Routledge and Kegan Paul, London 1981

Grills, J. and M. *Drug Abuse*, Oxford University Press, Oxford 1986

Higgins, J. *The Business of Medicine: Private Health Care in Britain*, Macmillan, London 1988

Illich, I. *Medical Nemesis*, Marion Boyars, London 1975

Inglis, B. *Natural Medicine*, Collins, London 1979 (this contains a useful list of addresses of organisations)

Lacey, R. and Woodward, S. *That's Life! Survey on Tranquillisers*, BBC, London 1985

LeGrand, J. *Open University Course D210 block 5 units 18 and 19*, Open University Press, Milton Keynes 1985

LeGrand, J. *The Strategy of Equality*, Allen and Unwin, London 1982

Mann, F. *Acupuncture: Cure of Many Diseases*, Pan Books, London 1973 (first published 1971)

Mathews, R. *Decarceration and the Fiscal Crisis*, in Fine, B. *et al*, (eds), *Capitalism and the Rule of Law*, Hutchinson, London 1979

Observer Modern Studies Handbook, *Drugs*, Observer, London 1986

Pinchuck, T. and Clark, R. *Medicine for Beginners*, Writers and Readers, London 1984

Robertson, R. *Heroin, AIDS and Society*, Hodder and Stoughton, London 1987

Salmon, J. W. *Alternative Medicines: Popular and Policy Perspectives*, Tavistock, London 1984

Scull, A. *Decarceration: Community Treatment and the Deviant, A Radical View*, Polity Press, London 1984 (first published 1977)

Stanway, A. *Alternative Medicine: A Guide to Natural Therapies*, Penguin, Harmondsworth 1986 (second edition)—has a good bibliography

Thomson, D. *The Overpaid Elderly?*, New Society, 7 March 1986

Tinker, A. *The Elderly in Modern Britain*, Longman, London 1984 (second edition)

Weitz, M. *Health Shock*, David and Charles, Newton Abbot 1980

Wells, N. and Freer, C. (eds), *The Ageing Population: Burden or Challenge?*, Macmillan, London 1988

Williams, M. *The Thatcher Generation*, New Society, 21 February 1986

Young, J. *The Role of the Police as Amplifiers of Deviancy*, in Cohen, S., (ed), *Images of Deviance*, Penguin, Harmondsworth 1971

The addresses of some of the organisations involved in alternative medicine are:

Society for the Promotion of Natural Health
Frazer House
6 Netherhall Gardens
London NW3
01 435 8728

The Vegan Society
47 Highlands Rd
Leatherhead
Surrey
03723 72389

British Homeopathic Association
27a Devonshire St
London
WIN IRJ
01 935 2163

The Chiropractic Advancement Association
38 The Island
Thames Ditton
Surrey
01 398 2098

Festival for Mind-Body-Spirit
159 George St
London
WI
01 723 7256

The Q Directory
17 Wolseley Rd
London
N8
01 348 4178

ASH
27–35 Mortimer St
London
WIN 7RJ

National Council on Alcoholism
3 Grosvenor Crescent
London
SW1 7EL

See *The Times* 14 August 1985 for a report on trials of
alternative therapies

Answers to *Drugwise* exercise, page 118: (each set of
three numbers refers to columns 1, 2 and 3 respectively)

1, 12, 3 (legal)
2, 10, 1 (illegal unless prescribed)
3, 11, 2 (illegal)
4, 9, 11 (legal)
5, 7, 10 (illegal unless prescribed)
6, 8, 12 (legal but only available on prescription)
7, 5, 8 (illegal)
8, 6, 9 (legal unless made into a preparation)
9, 4, 7 (illegal)
10, 1, 6 (illegal unless prescribed)
11, 2, 5 (illegal to sell to anyone under 16)
12, 3, 4 (legal to buy over 18 to use at any age over five
away from licensed premises)

For information on drugs, particularly a very useful
booklet called *Drug Abuse Briefing*, write to:
The Institute for the Study of Drug Dependence
1 Hatton Place
London
EC1N 8ND

The exercise on p. 118 is based on parts of the *Drugwise*
pack, available from the above address.

General Bibliography

Doyal, L. with Pennell, I., *The Political Economy of Health*, Pluto Press, London 1979

George, V. and Wilding, P., *Ideology and Social Welfare*, Routledge and Kegan Paul, London 1976

Graham, H., *Women, Health and the Family*, Wheatsheaf Books, London 1984

Hart, N., *The Sociology of Health and Medicine*, Causeway Press, Ormskirk 1985

LeGrand, J., *The Strategy of Equality*, Unwin Hyman, London 1982

Mishra, R., *Society and Social Policy*, Macmillan, London 1981 (2nd edition)

MacGregor, S., *The Politics of Poverty*, Longman, London 1981

Patrick, D. L. and Scambler, G., (eds), *Sociology as Applied to Medicine*, Balliere Tindall, Eastbourne 1986 (2nd edition)

Stacey, M., *The Sociology of Health and Healing*, Unwin Hyman, London 1988

Townsend, P., Davidson, N. and Whitehead, M., *Inequalities in Health*, Penguin, Harmondsworth 1988 (new edition, including *The Health Divide*)

Taylor-Gooby, P. and Dale, J., *Social Theory and Social Welfare*, Edward Arnold, London 1981

Walker, A. and Walker, C., *The Growing Divide*, Child Poverty Action Group, London 1987

Subject Index

Author Index

Acknowledgements

The author and publishers would like to thank the following:

for permission to reproduce text extracts and diagrams;

Basil Blackwell for the material from *The History of Medicine* by L. Hartley (p. 8, p. 58).

Questions 14–18 of Townsend's questionnaire taken from *Poverty in the United Kingdom* P. Townsend, reproduced by permission of Penguin Books Ltd (p. 35).

Oxford University Press, for two tables from R. Doll and R. Peto's *The Causes of Cancer*, 1980 (p. 39).

The Fabian Society for tables C, F, R, S, U from *The New A–Z of Income and Wealth* by T. Stark (pp. 47, 48, 53).

New Society for 'The Rich in Britain' extract, 22 August 1986, (p. 49), and a table from M. Williams's 'The Thatcher Generation', 21 February 1986, (p. 115).

The Open University for material from U221 unit 4 'The Changing Experience of Women' (p. 82–3).

for permission to reproduce illustrations;

Steve Bell p. 5, p. 103
GP Magazine, (Haymarket Publications) p. 21
Julia Martin (The Photo Co-op) p. 23
Keith Gibson p. 27
L. E. Bustamate (The Photo Co-op) p. 42
Ingrid Gavshon (The Photo Co-op) p. 42
Richard Branson and The Virgin Group PLC p. 54
Lawrence Greswell (The Photo Co-op) p. 64
The British Heart Foundation p. 68
The Health Education Authority p. 69
Maggie Murray (Format) p. 72
Gina Glover (The Photo Co-op) p. 79
Ronald Grant p. 85
Mencap p. 90
Spectrum p. 94
Brenda Prince (Format) p. 101
Raissa Page (Format) p. 103
New Society 6 February 1987, 'The Decade of Inequality' p. 109
BUPA p. 112